NOTICE

The information presented is not intended for the treatment or prevention of disease, as a substitute for medical treatment, or as an alternative to medical advice. **Please consult with a medical professional before beginning any training or supplement program.**

The publication is presented for informational and educational purposes. **Use of the information provided including the use of identified supplements is at the sole choice and the risk of the reader.**

This publication contains abstracts from a number of literature sources. These abstracts are provided for supplemental educational and informational purposes **only**, and in no way are intended to promote any position of the author. Moreover, the abstracts of their authors have not endorsed any supplement product identified in the publication, and the presentation of the abstracts should not be construed as doing so.

Any reprint or copying of this publication, whether in hard copy or electronically, is strictly prohibited without the express written permission of the author or his representatives.

Copyright 2008 Eric Marchewitz – All Rights Reserved

Table Of Contents

1) The Basics – Page 5

2) Protein & Amino Acids - Page 11

3) Creatine – 31

4) Beta Alanine NO Glutamine – 45

5) pSARMs, Herbals and Adaptagens – 57

6) Anti-Estrogens – 75

7) Prohormones – 95

8) Stimulants, Diet & GH Boosters – 115

9) Stacks & Cycles - 137

Copyright 2008

The Sports Supplement Guide

An article I recently read spawned the idea of writing a book about the basics of sports supplements. Those of you that read my previous book will know that it is possible to change your life and your genetics by simply taking the right sports supplements. For a young bodybuilder, it is hard to decide what products to use when starting and the natural progression of adding additional items to your supplement regimen to increase your response. This book will show you how to add the proper nutrients, the proper times to take them and the best way to add additional supplements to your arsenal to help you reach your goals of looking good and feeling even better.

Remember, you can feel free to skip around and mix and match the supplements in the pyramid. We will even give you some sample stacks to try.

THE BASICS

cGMP – Pick Quality Supplements

I must warn you of a very dangerous plague on the supplement industry. Did you know that unless a company uses GMP certified manufacturing, you have no way of knowing the quality and amount of the ingredients in your supplement and there is no control on what is actually in there?

Do you think I am kidding on how widespread this is? Without taking down the supplement industry and exposing myself to potential lawsuits, you the consumer, need to really insist on a new standard for supplements that ensures you fully receive what you pay for. This cGMP will be the law of the land very soon, but small companies (like those in the bodybuilding world) don't need to be cGMP compliant until 2010. The government (about one of the few things they are doing right) has issued mandatory GMP certification for dietary supplements, but it only covers a small segment of the market until all companies are required to comply, regardless of size, in 2010. I HIGHLY suggest you buy ONLY GMP certified today.

GMP is a federally imposed standard that assures quality and accuracy in your supplements. A word to the wise, buy ONLY GMP certified supplements.If you don't, there is no way to know what you are putting into your body. Trust only companies that use GMP certified labs to produce their supplement line in order to ensure that the product contains EXACTLY what is on the label. These supplements have been tested for purity and label integrity.

If you buy some off brand "bargain" supplement or products from a really small company, you could be getting saw dust for all you know, which means that you will not only waste time but money too! Look for GMP certification (on the bottle) for all of your supplements and nutritional needs. Don't think this doesn't happen. There are web sites specifically designed to expose supplement companies who do not meet label claims. Some of your most popular brands can test out to contain none of the ingredients that you THINK are in the bottle. Trust only the government GMP certification to ensure quality.

Bad ingredients make their way to the U.S. all the time. This stuff happens! Just look at the recent issues with pet food. In case you didn't follow it, pet food made with Chinese protein was killing innocent pets. The innocent U.S. manufacturers had no idea why this was happening until they tested some brands and found that the protein was "contaminated" with something that made it weigh more, making the protein more profitable for the Chinese suppliers yet hurt the pets. Why would Chinese manufacturers do this? Well, if the additive weighs more in the same volume yet costs less, they can charge the same for including less protein in their shipment. This stuff happens and the only remedy in the U.S. is GMP certification. I STRONGLY encourage you to look for a GMP logo on every supplement you purchase. If not, you may, at best, be throwing your money down the drain or, worse, putting something harmful into your body!

Vitamins, Minerals and Water...

Bodybuilders need supplements more than the average person because we put such a heavy burden on our bodies daily. Also, we may tend to drift into anabolics (whether legal or illegal) that carry some pretty heavy side effects. So, what is a good vitamin regimen for the average bodybuilder? The following is a list of the best supplements a bodybuilder should take, in order of importance.

There are three basic supplements you should strongly consider. Firstly, you want to take a GOOD multivitamin. Just because it comes in a pack doesn't mean that it is good. Find one from a reliable health food store and have them suggest a good one. MAKE SURE IT DOESN'T CONTAIN IRON IF YOU ARE A MAN! The minerals should contain chelates, such as magnesium chelate, not oxides or carbonates. These chelates are much more expensive but have the positive absorption that is necessary for a good multi. Along with these chelated minerals, make sure it has a high dose of Vitamin C and solid doses of everything you need. Secondly, you need to take a good Vitamin E product, not something in the value isle at your grocery store. Vitamin E has advanced past what you get in a supermarket, there is a new version of vitamin E called High Gamma E. I am not going to explain how it works, just understand that it is a much better form of vitamin E. The third, and perhaps most important, basic supplement for good health is a solid Fish Oil supplement. Fish Oil is amazing and protects your heart, liver and brain from damage and decay. You can't take just one though and expect to see any benefit. Fish Oil is cheap and you need to take at least 6 gel caps per day. Fish oil won't get you huge, but it will keep you healthy. I take 6-8 fish oil capsules per day with meals to help keep my omega 3 fats in good supply!

Now that we have the basics covered, we can move on to more exotic supplements for anti-aging and joint repair. CoQ10 is an enzyme co-factor that is great for keeping your heart and brain healthy and is, overall, a very good supplement for anyone interested in anti-aging (30-100mg per day). ALA or Alpha Lipoic Acid is even better because this anti-oxidant is also used by body builders to make insulin more active! It actually acts like some prescription insulin potentiators, which is a fancy way of saying it makes insulin more effective at carrying nutrients into your body (200-500mg per day with meals).

Don't underestimate the value of healthy joints, which is why ALL bodybuilders should take a good Glucosamine and Chondroiton supplement. Watch out for those that use Glucosamine HCL instead of Glucosamine Sulfate. You want Glucosamine Sulfate, since that Sulfur molecule is necessary and it is the form all positive studies have used. Although HCL is cheaper, it doesn't seem to offer the same benefit. There is nothing sadder than seeing an older bodybuilder that hasn't kept his joints in good health.

Also, drink plenty of Pomegranate juice (also available as a supplement, just DO NOT get the one with ellagic acid) for the health benefits, especially if you take steroids. Don't just pick any of them off the shelf, many are "cut" with grape juice, which is empty carbs. What will this do for you? Well, it shrinks the prostate, cleans clogged arteries and reduces oxidation in the body. It's truly the drink of champions and NECESSARY for bodybuilders that take anabolic steroids or anyone that wants to be healthy. There is no amount of money that can replace a healthy body, so make sure you budget for some good supplements in your quest to get huge!

Finally, people underestimate the value of water. Drinking at least one gallon of water per day will keep your system flushed and full. Water is a very important nutrient and a good solid program of one to one and a half gallons of water per day.

First Base: Protein and Amino Acids

Protein is the foundation for building muscle. The body cannot make it's own amino acids for muscle building, which means your protein will have to come from dietary sources every hour for maximum muscle growth. Proteins can come from many sources including animal and vegetable protein. Both animal and vegetable proteins make excellent sources and they both have their advantages and disadvantages. The bodybuilder should get between 1g and 2g of protein per pound of bodyweight. Meat of almost any kind (beef, chicken or fish) contains about 7g of protein per 1oz serving. A 4oz Chicken Breast will have 28g of protein. Cottage Cheese has 7g of protein per ¼ cup so it makes an excellent snack. Eggs also contain about 7g of protein each, so a hard boiled egg is also a good way to get extra protein. Supplement with a good protein shake too, just remember to eat BIG!

Animal proteins can come from food sources like chicken, fish, beef, pork, eggs and lamb. Animal proteins are complete proteins, meaning that they contain all of the essential amino acids needed for proper body growth. Unfortunately, animal proteins happen to have more fat and, in the case of beef, pork, and lamb, more cholesterol than their vegetarian counterparts. I happen to only eat kosher beef, which doesn't allow for the inhumane killing of animals and excludes pork. Although I am not Jewish, I do prefer to not harm animals as much as possible and certainly to limit their suffering. Animal proteins from non-organic sources can also contain high levels of pesticides, hormones and antibiotics. These things plus the disgusting conditions of animals in commercial farms make me stay away from animal sources except for the occasional kosher meal.

Eggs are also a good source of complete protein, yet the yolks contain cholesterol and a healthy dose of fat. This isn't always bad, but for the average person, cholesterol isn't the best thing for your heart. Eggs also make a good snack, but they tend to get old if they are your only source of protein.

Milk contains a fair amount of protein on its own, but it also includes pesticides, hormones and even some disgusting additives like puss and blood. Often, whitening agents are used in our milk to conceal their brownish color. After I read the impurities in milk along with the massive allergen quantity I have never had milk again. Drinking a glass, of puss, blood and allergy causing proteins isn't something that sounds too appealing, so I skip milk and milk-based proteins. However, milk does contain a good amount of sugar and protein and can be a good post workout drink.

Protein powders come in many flavors and from about as many sources. Protein powders can come as a complex of many types or as single proteins. Protein powders are different from weight gainers or meal replacement powders (MRP's) because they do not include extra sugar or fat. They usually don't taste as good as either MRP's or weight gainers, but then again you won't find that they contain large amounts of sugar either. Additionally, there are high fat based proteins that supposedly mimic milk, but they are just protein powders with extra fat and sugar, making them taste good but also high in calories. There are many types of protein in powdered drinks and the choices are endless in dietary consumer products. I will outline the most popular ones and their advantages and disadvantages.

Whey Protein Concentrate (WPC):
Whey is extracted from Milk and is a byproduct of cheese productions (eating her curds and whey). WPC usually comes in an 80% concentration, meaning that it is 80% protein. The other 20% is fat, lactose and moisture. The fat content of WPC is much higher than other proteins and the additional lactose makes many people bloated and gives the sick feeling often associated with protein shakes. WPC has many additional constituents that make it good for muscle growth and recovery. It is cited as a fast digesting protein and provides immediate amino acids for muscle repair. It is best used post-workout or in place of other high protein foods. WPC makes up most cheap proteins. I stay away from milk based proteins because of the high allergens and disgusting secondary ingredients, but if you have the stomach for that stuff, WPC is a good, cheap form of protein that works really well. Whey also contains high amounts of Branch Chain Amino Acids and Glutamine which are important for the bodybuilder.

Whey Isolate:
Whey Isolate contains the same positives as WPC, yet is a cleaner product with higher protein content. It usually contains very little fat and often zero lactose, which means it provides very little bloat. It is a complete protein that is quickly digested and is good substitute for WPC. Although it is far more expensive the cleaner feeling and lack of bloat makes whey isolate protein a better choice for the smart consumer. However, I also stay away from this milk-based protein due to the impurities and allergens explained above.

Milk Protein Isolate:
Milk protein Isolate is simply a raw blend of the milk proteins whey and casein. It is a good blend, but may have a slower absorption rate due to the casien, making it slightly less effective than straight whey. Since it is an isolate, it shouldn't cause much gas or bloating, but it does have the allergens from milk.

Calcium Caseinate:
Casein is another form of milk protein that takes longer to digest than whey. Calcium Caseinate is a synthetic extraction of casein from milk. Caseins tend to clump together in the stomach which makes them digest much more slowly than whey. There is some debate as to whether calcium caseinate is a good absorbable protein, but it should be similar to other to other caseinates and should provide a slow digesting complete protein source.

Micellar Casein:
This is a high price and higher quality casein-based protein. Like above, it is a slower digesting protein that supplies amino acids in a steady fashion. It has been shown to be not as anabolic as whey, but is still a viable source for protein. The problem with most casein is that it doesn't taste good. Micellar Casein is a good source of protein, but it doesn't mix well and tastes lousy compared to whey or other types of protein.

Egg Protein:
Egg protein is either derived from whole eggs or egg whites. The whole egg version has cholesterol and fat, which makes it undesirable for many bodybuilders. Egg white protein is a

much better form, but it tends to cost a bit more. Egg protein is a good source of protein for many bodybuilders and the old school guys will swear by egg as their favorite protein source. Egg protein tends to taste good to me, but it can have a sulphuric effect for many bodybuilders (i.e. smelly gas), which makes it unpleasant.

Soy Protein:
Soy is technically an incomplete protein, meaning it lacks one essential amino acid. Soy also has isoflavones that can be considered estrogenic. This isn't a big deal to me, but many people fear the estrogenic effects of soy along with it possibly messing with T3 levels. Soy is a good source of protein for supplemental intake, since you will need to make up that missing amino acid from other protein sources. Soy isn't very popular with bodybuilders these days because of its flavones and amino acid profile.

Genus Protein:
Genus protein is the newest protein on the market. It is a complete protein that is even higher in protein content than whey, branch chain amino acids and glutamine. It is very low in fat and carbohydrates yet remains high in complete amino acids. This is the best protein source for the bodybuilder looking to supplement their protein intake without extra carbs and fat (one serving has less than 1g of carbohydrate and less than 1g of fat). This makes Genus protein the most amazing protein source in the past 10 years. This new protein source should take the industry by storm once people get their hands on it. Genus has one other unique characteristic, it contains fat burning polyphenols that are similar to the anti-oxidant

polyphenols in green tea. This makes Genus protein the best source of protein for someone looking to build muscle while burning fat. Genus is an up and coming protein; look for it in many newer formulations.

Collagen Based Protein:
Collagen protein is extracted from the hooves, cartilage and joints of pigs and cattle. It is a pretty low grade protein over all, but it does provide a good boost in protein that is convenient. Ordinarily Collagen protein isn't used in bodybuilding (basically being just "Jell-o") because it isn't terribly complete as a protein source, but for someone that is looking to increase total dietary intake in a very convenient manner, collagen does the trick. Better grades of collagen are nearly flavorless and colorless, making them attractive packaging for the average person who wants somethibvng tasty and convenient. Sometimes collagen is mixed with other proteins to increase its nutrient profile, which can help make it a better source of protein for the person on the go.

Hydrolyzed Proteins:
Proteins can be hydrolyzed, which means broken into smaller pieces or semi-digested. Soy, whey and collagen are commonly hydrolyzed proteins. Unfortunately, hydrolyzed proteins taste like utter horror, so they are rarely used in protein formulations. However, hydrolyzed proteins provide one huge benefit over standard undigested proteins. Hydrolyzed proteins absorb much more quickly and hit the blood stream faster than any other form of protein. Often, you will find hydrolyzed proteins being sold as amino acids, but you should stay away from such formulas, since hydrolyzed

proteins are not the same as free form amino acids. Hydrolyzed proteins usually form large polypeptides, which are faster absorbing than straight protein but still not the same as a mix of free form amino acids. Still, post workout hydrolyzed proteins offer a good way to slam some serious anabolic building blocks right into your muscle.

"Milk" Analogs:
There is a trend in the industry to attempt mimicking the effects of "Milk" by blending a lot of low quality fats and sugars into your protein in order to make them taste good. These blends often promote the fats as being "leaner" than other fats, which is simply not true. Soybean and canola oil are not any leaner than any other type of fats. Maltodextrin is used in place of sugar in an attempt to reduce the glycemic index (GI), which is a joke. Maltodextrin may be a lower GI sugar, but it tastes horrible, doesn't help you lose any fat weight or do anything positive for the average bodybuilder. My advice is to skip these proteins. Anything with over 12g of sugar per serving and the nutrient profile of a Big Mac isn't going to be good for you. Sure, they taste great, but if you are looking for taste, just get that Big Mac, it will be more satisfying and if you take a scoop of low fat protein with it, provide the same nutrient profile. You should skip these "Milk" based proteins completely and use something lean and mean like Whey or Genus.

What is the best overall protein?

That is a tough question, but overall whey is proven and well known in the body building world as the standard on which all other proteins are judged. However new contenders like Genus Protein certainly offer some unique benefits over whey and look like the up and comers. Many old school bodybuilders prefer egg protein, but the reality is that protein should come from a variety of sources and no one is really the "best". The average person looking to supplement for maximum effect should take 1-2 g of protein per pound of body weight, meaning that a 200 lb male should take between 200 and 400 grams of protein per day. Meat contains about 7g of protein per ounce, no matter what the source, so look for lean cuts of beef, chicken As long as you are eating lean chicken, fish, beef, lamb or buffalo you should be able to get some serious protein from meat. If you are a humegitarian like me (only eating animals from hunted or kosher sources which limits the animals suffering and/or helps it fulfill its life potential) a good protein supplement is essential.

Meals and timing:

Here is my recommendation for the optimal protein regimen for the average bodybuilder wishing to gain maximum size and recovery:

Breakfast – Clean protein sources like egg whites provide good breakfast proteins and some nice variety. You can also cook some lean beef along with your egg whites to add additional protein or throw in 1 cup of cottage cheese to your breakfast, adding in 28g of protein to your diet.

Midmorning Shake – Genus Protein provides the optimal nutrient profile without adding in a lot of extra fat or calories.

Also, the polyphenols in Genus protein stoke the metabolic furnace, which gives you the optimal mid-morning shake. Around 10:00 AM is the best time to use your Genus protein.

Lunch – obviously lunch proteins can include chicken breast, turkey or any other lean source of protein along with some complex carbohydrates.

Mid-afternoon Shake – Again, use Genus protein for its fat burning and high amino acid profile.

Post-Workout – Any sort of hydrolyzed protein will do, including free form amino acids or collagen protein. This will rapidly feed your muscles with the optimal dose of fast hitting proteins to refuel your muscle. Take with 20-30g of dextrose (stay away from Corn Syrup) or other sugars for maximum effect.

Dinner – Lean beef or fish make excellent choices.

Before Bed – Use Miceller Casein or Sodium Caseinate to give you long-acting proteins for the night's sleep. Micellar Casein is a nice, slow digesting protein that will feed your body with the necessary amino acids to give you recovery and growth.

The bottom line on protein is GET LOTS OF IT. You can get really fancy about the types of protein you are going to take and, for the elite athlete, it matters. However, most people should just go with a straight protein shake like Genus to provide the additional protein needed without breaking the bank.

Protein mixes that combine egg, whey, casein and others are just gimmicks. If you want to use proteins like that positively, time them according to when they are needed. Throwing them all in a blend isn't going to get you anything special and they usually cost MUCH more.

Bars...the good, the fat and the false!

Bars are quite a funny phenomenon over the years, transforming from sugar laden high-calorie treats, to barely edible bricks, to falsely labeled delectables and finally nutritional abortions that taste really good!

Back in the 80's, bars like the "Steel" bar and others tasted great but had a ton of sugar and corn syrup in order to give them an almost candy bar type appearance. They tasted good, but their nutrient profile was lacking for anyone but the most intense hard gainer that needed calories more than nutrition. After the Atkins revolution, we were served up some horrible tasting bars that claimed ZERO sugar and ZERO carbs, which the FDA ultimately called misleading. These bars contained high amounts of glycerin, which is a high calorie slow digesting sugar like molecule. It was claimed to be zero carb, because it doesn't spike insulin, but it was shown to still take you out of ketosis, which means that those calories mattered!

After some time, the labels changed on these bars and a new crop of "mislabeled" bars came into existence. The first one appeared as a Semi-Snickers bar. I remember taking a detour into my friends shop to get one of these beauties. They claimed low sugar, low calories, but were oozing with caramel and tasted like a snickers. I remember Frank commenting "Isn't that the greatest bar you have ever tasted? Something is up...". A few months later reports started to surface about the bar being mislabeled and some inquiries were made. Oddly enough, I picked up one of these bars are Frank's place in Detroit and guess what...no more caramel, no more taste...more calories? What happened? Well, when something is too good to be true, it often is... These bars were found to contain more fat and sugar than reported and the manufacturer quickly replaced them with "truer" bars that tasted like crap. Sadly, this company is still on the market making lousy tasting glycerin bars.

The second "Fako Bar" came out about a year later. A 400lb Chef thought that he could make a better bar for the bodybuilding community and he released several flavors of his bar, which was a monstrosity that had 360 calories. I tried the Apple Caramel at Franks, and it was moist and flavorful with soft pieces of apple and big chunks of caramel. Soon, some inquiries were made into the label claims on these bars and I happened to have one a few months later. The calories ballooned to 460 calories and when I bit into the bar, the soft gooey caramel was replaced by a rock hard brick that tastes like a gut busting cement bar. What happened? How did we add 100 calories yet lose so much in taste, texture and flavor?

Welcome to the world of sports supplements, where you can put anything on the label you want and no one knows the better... I only buy supplements from GMP certified manufacturers, which ensures that all of the ingredients are in there and that the product actually meets label claims.

Finally, the industry sort of grew up. Taking advantage of our American "we don't care" lifestyle, a host of new bars are on the market that taste great, but contain the nutritional profile of an average fast food meal. Sure, they have 25g of protein, but most of them have over 25g of sugars and over 14g of fat. Check your local fast food joint and you will see that you can get better than that from a chicken sandwich without mayo!

I am not a fan of bars for everyday use. As a meal replacement, they are fine occasionally, but as a protein supplement, you can do WAY better by getting a good shake or a small cottage cheese.

Amino Acids... not all are equal

Nine amino acids are generally regarded as essential for humans: phenylalanine, valine, threonine, tryptophan, isoleucine, methionine, histidine, leucine, and lysine. Also, the amino acids arginine, cysteine, glycine, glutamine, and tyrosine are considered conditionally essential, meaning they are not normally required in the diet but may have other uses that are good for humans. Beware of scam amino acid products. I bought some pretty expensive optimized amino acids with 2222 mg per serving, only to discover upon closer inspection that the main ingredient was just Soy Protein! What a scam, I just paid 14 bucks for soy protein in a capsule? This is an example of letting the buyer beware for sure and pretty scummy if you ask me. Amino Acids are NOT just protein, they are the building blocks of protein. Proteins come in things called peptide chains, which are links of amino acids that make up a protein. Proteins have many functions in the body as do singular amino acids. Unfortunately, taking in an amount of "protein" that contains 2000mg of X amino acid never seems to translate to the benefits that one can get by taking singular amino acids. This is a theory I have been working on for the past 14 years. My father had a book about manipulating your brain chemistry via amino acids and after reading that book, I was hooked! My love affair with Amino Acids was born. I have used amino acids to do everything from modulate my moods to heal tissue and certainly build muscle. I have also filed a novel patent pending on Amino Acids to create the world's first di-peptide singular amino acids for certain functions.

Amino acids differ from proteins in their ability to have a profound effect on multiple aspects of body chemistry. Taking a piece of beef with 1g of Arginine for example has little or no similarity to taking 1g of a singular Arginine Amino Acid. Taking singular amino acids can have such amazing effects and it is this mix of amino acid benefits that can make their use a real benefit to bodybuilders. I will discuss many of the singular aminos and amino acid derivatives in later chapters of this book but make no mistake, taking amino acids from full protein sources like beef or soy do not share much relationship to the singular amino acids found in supplements. Therefore, taking amino acids can really help the bodybuilder.

The aminos I am going to cover in this chapter, from a supplement perspective are broad spectrum predigested amino acids with a low peptide ratio. These are the hydrolyzed proteins that can be used to increase recovery. In later chapters, we will get into more specific amino acid blends and cocktails that have a broad range of effects. In this chapter however, I will detail each amino acid and define some basic functions that each amino can be used for medicinally. However, the bulk of the information will be about supplementing with amino acids as a mean of improving recovery.

The best time to take your amino acids is right after training. Best taken with a high sugar drink (I DIDN'T say corn syrup), amino acids can provide unique building blocks for muscle that can't be gotten with proteins alone. Taking hydrolyzed aminos gives you the quickest refeed possible for hungry muscle tissue. So, a good hydrolyzed protein and sugar mean after a workout is perfect for the bodybuilder looking to maximize gains. Also, amino acids and a sugar drink prior to any performance activity is the best way to ensure proper energy production and muscle effects. These are often combined with one of the insulin potentiators or mimetics on the market like Chromium Picolinate or Vanadyl Sulfate or both. This powerful cocktail is a good way to grind out more reps, run just a little longer or increase your best time on the bike. Amino Acid drinks and shots give the power lifter, trained athlete or bodybuilder the extra push and energy needed to get the most out of each workout. Luckily, they are light on the stomach and are usually fairly tasty (depending upon the sources). Hydrolyzed Collagen/Whey blends mixed with water and sugar make a good drink to sip on while you are performing your sets. Make sure you get predigested hydrolyzed proteins so you don't waste any energy on digestion when it should be going towards running, jumping or push/pull

type activities.
Branched Chain Amino Acids (BCAA):

Leucine, Isoleucine and Valine are called Branch Chain Amino Acids. These are the amino acids that are actually anabolic in muscle. The real heavy lifter here seems to be L-Leucine. Leucine has been shown to be anabolic in muscle on its own and has an amazing ability to help recovery. It has been shown to reduce muscle breakdown, increase anabolism and is even implicated in burning fat! This wonder amino acid is part of a cascade of amino acids that are really important to building muscle. Unfortunately, Leucine is conditionally dependent on the other branched chain aminos, so it is important to get all three. There is some debate however on how much of all three you need to be effective. The generally accepted ratios are not really necessary, I would take a BCAA product and spike it with a 1:1 ratio with straight L-Leucine powder to get the maximum effect. If you are taking plenty of quality protein, you are getting enough of the supportive Isoleucine and Valine to reduce the negative effects of straight Leucine supplementation. This in addition to straight protein is the most important nutrient that you can take to increase metabolism of new muscle cells. Supplement 3-5g of BCAA's prior to working out and another 3-5g right after your workout to get maximum effects.

A great recipe for performance would be:
Honey + Distilled Water
Hydrolyzed Whey or BCAA's

Extra Leucine:
This cocktail would really put the hurt on any known sports drink or formula on the market. Most drinks (especially in the U.S.) are actually counterproductive. Unfortunately, with the cheapness of corn, the modern U.S. diet is filled with High Fructose Corn Syrup. This became a staple in most American formulations, not because of nutritional benefit, but because corn syrup is cheap and easy to store. Corn Syrup has been implicated in the rising obesity rates in the U.S. and the high incidents of diabetes due to it not having the same level of satiety that sugar contains (it doesn't make you full). This might be why you can suck down a large coke and still eat another 1200 calories from the value menu, while our European counterparts eat far smaller portions and feel full. Honey, is a good, proven energy source and the perfect carrier for our hydrolyzed proteins. You can just buy an off the shelf protein shot (many exist, one unique one is in a resealable pouch with 45g per serving) mix it with your honey, water and the leucine if you have it and GO...

This is the absolute best way to supplement your diet with amino acids for muscle growth. Ordinarily, protein is digested slowly and adequately for repair. However, to maximize growth and repair, the best time to ingest your amino acids is during and immediately after your workout.

Liver Tabs – These are pretty useless amino acid containing items. Liver has some nutrients and amino acids but is also the filtering point for toxins which are really not good to put back into the body! Liver has a decent amino acid profile I guess, but it really isn't going to add anything to your body's ability to put on muscle. Liver tabs are something that should die and go away, but it is one of those legacy products that just won't die...

The Common Amino Acids

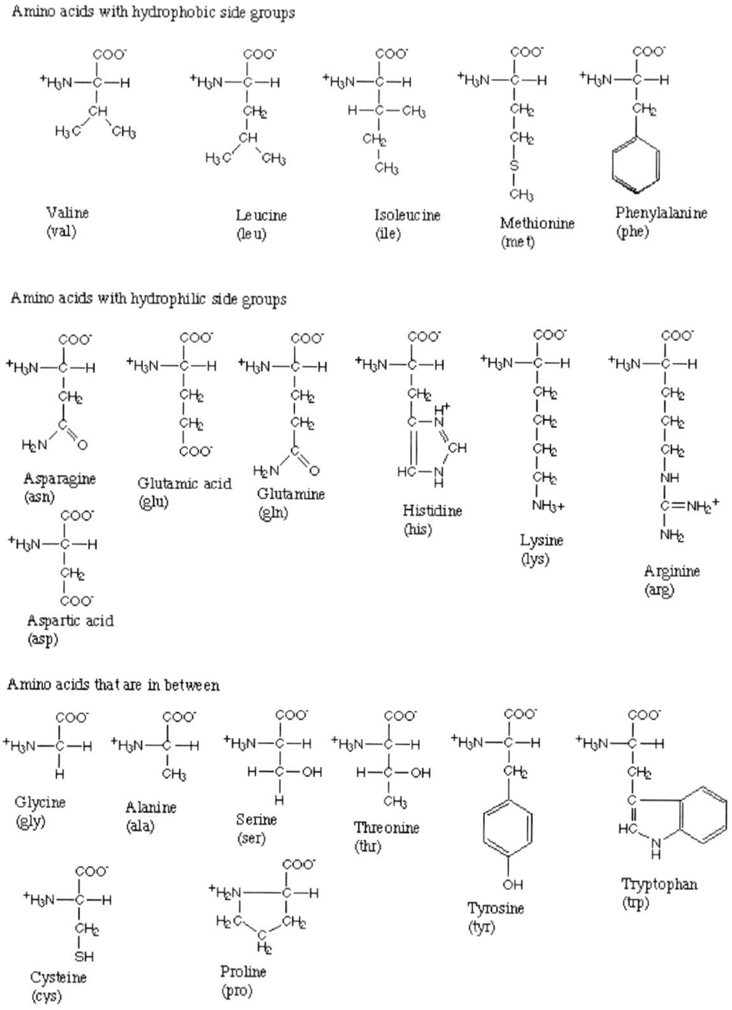

Amino acids with hydrophobic side groups

Valine (val), Leucine (leu), Isoleucine (ile), Methionine (met), Phenylalanine (phe)

Amino acids with hydrophilic side groups

Asparagine (asn), Glutamic acid (glu), Glutamine (gln), Histidine (his), Lysine (lys), Arginine (arg)

Aspartic acid (asp)

Amino acids that are in between

Glycine (gly), Alanine (ala), Serine (ser), Threonine (thr), Tyrosine (tyr), Tryptophan (trp)

Cysteine (cys), Proline (pro)

RANKING INDEX

Protein:

Genus Protein	******
Whey Isolate	******
Whey Concentrate	*****
Egg Protein	*****
Milk Protein	*****
Micellar Casein	*****
Calcium Caseinate	****
Collagen Protein	***
Soy Protein	***
High Fat "MILK" blends	**

Amino Acid Supplements:

High Luceine BCAA	******
BCAA	*****
Essential Amino Acids	*****
Hydrolyzed Proteins	****
Liver Tabs	***
Fake Amino Acid (just protein)	*

Bottom line:

- Take 1-2g per pound of lean body weight of protein per day from a variety of sources.
- Beef, fish, chicken, turkey, eggs, Genus protein and others make some of the best sources for daily supplementation.
- Cottage cheese or micellar casein is best right before bed for all night muscle feeding.
- Protein bars are often filled with fat and sugar and are only to be used as a treat.
- Amino acid drinks can be a huge benefit immediately after a workout, but be careful what you buy, since many purported amino acid complexes are nothing but soy or whey protein in a capsule or powder.
- BCAA's with extra leucine provide the best recovery agent and anabolic activator.

Creatine – The Proven Champion Of Sports Supplements

With all of the choices out there, how can we decide what is the best form of creatine, if such a thing actually does exist. Creatine is an amino acid that is naturally occurring in the body and provides cellular energy and a host of other benefits to both the bodybuilder and general health enthusiast. In fact, creatine is even being looked at to provide increased energy and wellness benefits for the elderly. It may provide heart benefits and may also increase mental acuity for people that have diseases such as Alzheimer's. Creatine is responsible for turning ADP into ATP, which is your body's main energy supply in the mitochondria. ATP is split to form ADP (losing a phosphate to create energy) and Creatine Phosphate "hangs around" to recharge the ADP molecule so it can be used to create energy again. Any Creatine is converted to Creatine Phosphate in the body, but oddly enough taking Creatine Phosphate as a supplement never really gave the kind of results that were achieved by many other creatine types, so it was effectively scrapped. Creatine is the base product for any bodybuilder looking to increase size and strength. It adds well to any other product and the only thing more basic than creatine is a protein supplement. Creatine helps the muscle cell hold more water, which can expand the fascia of the muscle increasing its volume. So, creatine is useful for strength and stamina by recharging the muscle energy system. It also increases new muscle cells, monohydrate for sure, and increases pumps for a muscle stretching effect. It is the most popular and beneficial supplement ever for bodybuilders.

The Structure Of Creatine:

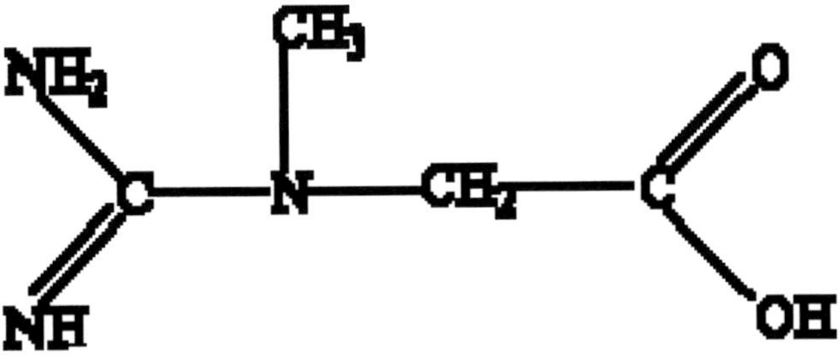

```
    CH₃
NH₂  |         O
  \\  |         ‖
   C—N—CH₂—C
  //            \
 NH              OH
```

Here is a basic list of just some of the Creatines on the market:

Creatine Monohydrate – This is the original version sold back in the 80's for improving strength and stamina for weightlifters;it is tried and tested. However, it has been replaced with newer and fancier creatine molecules. I HIGHLY suggest supplements still contain some creatine monohydrate for one big reason. Creatine Monohydrate is the only form proven in scientific studies to create new muscle cells. There are many studies showing Creatine Monohydrate increases the formation of new muscle cells and one important study showing that other forms of creatine do not have this effect!

Creatine DiPeptide – This is the most recent advance in creatine supplements. Creatine Dipeptides give all of the advantages of Creatine Monohydrate, with improved stability and increased absorption. This latest advance should provide the next level of creatine supplementation, yet still provide the benefits of the creatines of old.

Creatine Malate – This is creatine bound to malic acid. The preferred form is DiCreatine Malate since that is the only form that is possible. The other forms (Tricreatine Malate) are usually just creatine monohydrate mixed with straight malic acid. The supposed benefit of Creatine Malate is reduced bloating and increased endurance, since malate is involved in increasing cellular energy by being part of the Krebs cycle. Overall, this ingredient has many years of solid anecdotal support and is a good addition to any creatine blend. DO NOT BUY TRICREATINE MALATE-BASED PRODUCTS. This molecule is proven to NOT exist, so you really don't know what you are getting with this supplement.

Creatine Aspartate – This is creatine bound to aspartic acid. This is very similar to Creatine Malate and should prove to be even better for endurance athletes, since aspartate is even more directly involved in recharging the mitochondrial energy system. Creatine Aspartate is an improved form of Creatine Malate, but both should give very good endurance gains without extra bloat.

Creatine Ethyl Ester HCL – The latest "big splash" is Creatine Ethyl Ester. This ingredient has some strong anecdotal evidence of it working, but the science behind it is very flawed. The "ester" is supposed to make the creatine more absorbable and fat soluble. This belief is pretty flawed since creatine dissolves quite easily in water and there is little chance of it becoming fat soluble with this ester even if it was desirable to do so. Most likely, this product works by stabilizing the Creatine molecule with the HCL portion, which slows down some of the conversion to creatine (a waste product). Recently three landmark studies have been released showing Creatine Ethyl Ester to not perform as well as creatine monohydrate and creatine salts, like creatine malate. These studies show a very low conversion to biological creatine and very little conversion to the parent creatine molecule.

Creatine Gluconate – This product is simply creatine bonded to either sugar or glucose. No idea why that would be a big advantage over dumping some sugar in with your monohydrate, but it certainly doesn't hurt anything. Sugar helps the uptake of creatine in the cell, so it could have a positive effect.

Creatine Decanoate – I have no clue why anyone would want to bond decanoic acid to creatine unless they just want to take advantage of the "deca" in the name. Decanoic acid doesn't seem to increase performance or provide any benefits and this is probably a really bad idea in a supplement.

Creatine AKG – This is simply creatine bound to alpha keto glutarate, which is a glutamine type molecule. There is no real data on this ingredient but, in theory, it should work pretty well since both creatine and glutamine are good for you. AKG should help with the absorption of creatine, so this is a preferred form of creatine and a good addition to a creatine supplement.

Creatine Magnesium Chelate – This is another creatine molecule bound to magnesium. Chelated minerals were very popular as a way of increasing the absorption. There is certainly nothing wrong with magnesium, since it is great for you, but I don't see the positive benefit of binding creatine to a mineral when you could just take a good magnesium supplement and plain old monohydrate. Still, it isn't a bad idea since people can always benefit from more magnesium in their diet.

Creatine Orotate – Similar to Creatine Malate and Creatine Aspartate, Creatine Orotate provides increases cellular energy and improves absorption. Orotic acid benefits the bodybuilder by increasing strength and stamina. So the addition of orotic acid to creatine should yield some great benefits over other forms of creatine.

Creatinol-O-Phosphate - This is technically not creatine, but it is often lumped in with creatine products. This ingredient has some very good science behind it for increasing endurance and buffering lactic acid. It's not really a replacement for creatine but should work well in conjunction with it. It's ability to buffer lactic acid, increase work capacity and potentially enhance workload makes this ingredient look really good as an addition to creatine and beta alanine.

Well, that is a short list of the types of creatines that are on the market. A mixed form of multiple creatines is the best way to take a creatine supplement. I would, for sure, have some Creatine Monohydrate with your other mixes, since, as stated above, only Creatine Monohydrate is proven in scientific literature to actually increase satellite cells (new muscle growth). Whereas, some of the other products like Creatine Malate d0 not have this effect. Without new muscle cells, a bodybuilder can only get so big, which is why some people are "hard gainers".

So, how do you decide on the best creatine for you? A mix of different creatine types is probably a good idea to cover all of the bases. Then, add good supportive nutrients that give your desired effect. Insulin potentiators are certainly a good idea since they were the first real advance in creatine supplementation. Popular creatine potentiators are momodica (momordica) or bitter melon, cinnamon extract, alpha lipoic acid and 4-hydroxy-isolucine. These all help shove more material into the cells including creatine. Also, find one with some pharmaceutical grade dextrose in it. Most companies use Maltodextrin, which is totally useless for this and also tastes bad! Stay away from Maltodextrin-based supplements because they do nothing but add extra calories. Pharmaceutical Dextrose, however, provides a natural insulin spike and helps the potentiators do their job.

Creatine has been proven in multiple studies, and real-world experiences, to give the performance athlete benefits in increased muscle size, strength and performance. It is extremely safe, with over ten years of use. There is a limit, however, as to how much a bodybuilder should take. For example, anything over 20g of creatine per day could actually be counter-productive and even using that level should always be done during a loading phase for a maximum of 5 days. Also, for safety and efficacy, creatine should be cycled for up to 12 weeks, before taking one to two weeks off. This ensures that the body doesn't adapt to the higher levels. This isn't a proven method, but is just probably a good idea. Creatine can genetically alter your physique (see my previous book – *Never be small again...changing your genetics with sports supplements*) by increasing the amount of satellite cells, making it one of the most useful supplements ever invented.

Many things have been alleged about creatine over the years, from "steroids" to causing kidney damage. None of these allegations have ever panned out and creatine is considered safe and effective by the hundreds of thousands of people that use it daily as a means of increasing their performance. Creatine is also very good for elderly people who tend to lose muscle mass easily and consistently over time. I give my mother and father creatine daily as a way to help them keep muscle and brain functions at optimal levels.

Things Commonly Added To Creatine:

Waxy Maize Starch

This is a cool starch that actually helps draw water and creatine into the muscle cells. It seems to work really well at providing volumization according to anecdotal reports. There are several variants of this starch out there, but it is pretty good for increasing the potential of creatine and helping you feel "full", which, let's face it, is why people loved creatine from the start. Still, this is just another carb source that is slowly metabolized into muscle sugar, not anything revolutionary.

Glycocyamine

This is sort of the precursor to creatine. It has been used for many years now and, quite honestly, it doesn't seem to do much past what regular creatine will do for you and has a lesser effect. It has also been alleged to cause damage to other tissues and increase damaging proteins in the body.

Accordingly, it will often have betaine included to help quench the cellular proteins that cause damage and reduce ROS levels. Probably isn't a good thing to have in your creatine since it seems to be just a lot of money for nothing and can increase homocystine levels.

Guanidino Propionic Acid (GPA)
GPA can be used in creatine formulations to help increase insulin sensitivity and also provides some ergogenic benefit on its own. GPA has been shown to cause some damage to tissues though because it reduces cellular energy output (the opposite of what creatine does). This makes it pretty useful for weightloss but is, logically, counter-productive with creatine.

Alpha Lipoic Acid (ALA)
This helps increase insulin sensitivity and, along with sugar, helps bring creatine into the cell. It is a good ingredient that has a good place in those products that contain a lot of sugar.

4-Hydroxy-Isoleucine
This is an insulin mimetic that helps bring sugar and creatine into the muscle. Unlike ALA, which increases the sensitivity to insulin, this actually acts like insulin by shuttling sugar into the muscles.

Momordica
This extract of bitter melon is another insulin mimetic that shoves more nutrients into the muscle. It is a little better than the others out there since it shuttles both amino acids and sugars into the muscle. The other products just shuttle sugar into the muscle, so this has a big advantage.

Caffeine

You will find caffeine in many formulas to help increase the "feel" of the product. This isn't a good idea, but people do it to give you something that adds to the stimulation effect of a supplement.

D-Pinnitol

This is another insulin mimetic product that can increase the loading phase.

Cinnamon Extraction (Cinnulin PF (TM))

Cinnamon extract also has very good insulin mimetic effects that can be a good combination with creatine and sugars.

Peak ATP (TM)

This is literally ATP, the body's main energy source. Adenosine Tri Phosphate is broken down rapidly in the gut however, so little oral ATP, if any, gets into the blood stream. That being said, it can help by adding small amounts of Adinosine and Phosphates. ATP is charged by creatine during the cellular process. So, it isn't a bad idea to take some with your creatine. However, the amounts in sports supplements are not really enough to do anything positive in my opinion.

Liquid Serums

This is one of those products that just won't die, no matter what people do to kill it. The small amounts of creatine in there are pretty pointless and there is reason to believe that the creatine contained therein degrades quickly to inert ingredients. Like a bad email chain, this product will not go away since it tastes like fruit juice and looks like something cool and interesting. I would not buy these liquid creatine products no matter what.

IP6 – Inositol Hexaphospate
IP6 is simply the pseudo-vitamin Insitol with 6 phosphates bound to it. This is actually a really cool ingredient that adds additional benefits to creatine by supplying much needed phosphates along with IP6, which happens to be a pretty good ergogenic aid itself. The only downside to IP6 is its cost, which makes it tough to include enough to make it worthwhile for most creatine mixes.

Crazy Amino Acids - EX: Leucine Taurinate
These are simply just joining two amino acids and may or may not provide benefit over singular amino acids or peptides. These amino acids usually have no science behind them and are "feather dusted" into formulas to make them sound cool. Often these ingredients are just linking of two known amino acids in hopes that the interesting name will "wow" you. Peptides when designed correctly have a really good possibility of being better than the singular amino acids, but not when just thrown together to sound good in trace amounts. Creaine mixes may have quite a few ingredients, but if you need a microscope to read them, then they are probably nothing special.

Dextrose
This is just a common sugar that is very fast digesting. It's a fine energy source and should spike insulin and get "more" creatine into your system.

Maltodextrin
This is just a combination of Maltose and Dextrose. According to many experts, it isn't a very good carb source, since the

Maltose makes for a pretty unusable carb until it is further metabolized. There is information that shows that maltodextrin is a lower GI carb, which is why it is included in many formulas. Unfortunately, it is really not much better than sugar for reducing insulin load and is worse for replenishing carb sources. No idea why this became so popular except that it is one of those "urban legend" products.

RANKING INDEX

Creatine Peptides	******
Creatine Monohydrate	******
Creatine Orotate	*****
Creatine Malate	*****
Creatine Citrate	*****
Creatine Magnesium Chelate	*****
Creatine Gluconate	*****
Creatine AKG	*****
Creatine Ethyl Ester	**
Creatine Decanoate	**
Creatine Serums	*

Beta Alanine
NO Products
Glutamine

This level of the supplement pyramid contains ingredients to boost strength, recovery and nutrient delivery. These items are sometimes debatable and we will discuss the positives and negatives of such supplements and look at their use. Beta Alanine and these other items are very useful in many cases and we can look at their use, which has some very good support and also some negative reports.

Beta Alanine and Other Carnosine Boosters

This is a somewhat new item that was first introduced by MAN sports a few years ago. This item is now all the rage when it comes to sports supplements and you will be hard pressed to find a new creatine or NO blend without Beta Alanine. Luckily, Beta Alanine is as good as all the hype for increasing strength, stamina and recovery. Beta Alanine converts into muscle carnosine with the addition of Histdine (a very plentiful amino acid). Muscle carnosine can really increase strength and recovery through the recharging of anti-oxidants and direct reduction of H+ free radicals. The process of recharging ATP via creatine causes the production of H+ free radicals (hydrogen), which can cause muscle damage, increased aging and slower metabolism. Carnosine via Beta Alanine has been shown in numerous studies to reduce fatigue and increase the positive effects of creatine supplementation. This is probably the most exciting amino acid type nutrient to hit the market in many years.

Buffering lactic acid and other negative effects of exercise is the main method muscle carnosine and Beta Alanine work. It also seems to have a direct ergogenic aid besides being a buffer. The reported strength increases are unparalleled and Beta Alanine is implicated in many performance athletes' strength gains. The buffering of respiratory acids and radicals can have a profound effect on aging and cellular repair. This is one of the best anti-aging supplements on the market, so it is great for older people who wish to increase their lifespan.

The effective dose of Beta Alanine is 1500 – 2000mg per day. It can be taken all at once or in divided doses. However, it does have one down side when consumed, which is an itchy tingle that can be annoying. This tingle is caused by the stimulation of skin nerve cells in response to the higher beta alanine content. It feels like a niacin flush and lasts from 5-30 minutes. There is no reason to be alarmed by this flush but it can startle the person using Beta Alanine for the first time.

I think Beta Alainine is one of the key products in this slice of the pyramid and should be where you spend your supplement dollars once the basics like creatine and protein are budgeted. Luckily, you can find Beta Alanine in a mix of newer creatine products and, as long as you get over 1000mg per day, you can stack the two in one supplement. I would put Beta Alanine at the top of any supplement program.

Beta Alanine
This is the base product, an isomer of L-Alanine (not to be confused) that has the benefits discussed in the above article. Beta Alanine is well-absorbed and does not need these new fancy modifications to be active. It causes a flush type response as evidence of its efficacy and quick absorption. The flush response can actually happen in less than 5 minutes. The

only addition to Beta Alanine that could be useful is the addition of an insulin mimetic.

Beta Alanine Ethyl Ester
This is a hybrid product that jumps on the ethyl ester bandwagon. There is absolutely no data showing Ethyl Ester based amino acids does anything or has any advantage over the straight amino acid. In fact, the ethyl ester creates ethanol in the body and dilutes the amino acids that it is meant to help absorb. There is no reason to believe that the ethyl ester is good for anything and I would avoid these products since they are useless. Recently, it was shown that the body has a very limited ability to break these esters apart using esterase, which makes this a bad choice for someone wanting Beta Alanine.

Carnosine
This is just an expensive form of Beta Alanine since it rapidly degrades in the stomach into 60% Beta Alanine and 40% Histadine. It does have all the same benefits of Beta Alanine but is just far too expensive to use in a sports supplement. It is actually cheaper to just buy histadine and beta alanine and combine them. There is nothing wrong with Carnosine; it is just not very cost effective.

NO Boosters – Mixed Reviews...

The theory behind NO boosting agents is that they help the body open up its blood vessels and arteries to give better pumps and increase nutrient flow. There are mixed reviews on NO products though since they have been shown to not build much muscle in supplemented strength athletes. Like anything, one nutrient isn't going to help you, the bodybuilder reach all of your goals. It is only through the coupling of many agents that you can achieve your goals for strength and size. NO boosters have really gotten exotic over the years and each company likes to push the envelope on NO delivery and potentiators (things that increase NO).

NO stands for Nitric Oxide, which is a gas that is released in the many vessels and arteries in the body. This gas causes the arteries to relax and open up, which dilates them, causing increased blood flow. NO boosting agents are well known and the best known agent is Nitro Glycerine. This explosive is often given to heart patients to relax blood vessels and increase blood flow. The product is slipped under the tongue if any heart problems are sensed. NO boosting products like Arginine have also been shown to help burn fat and increase metabolism, so they are certainly good at producing a cut look in many ways.

The best known use of NO manipulation is in male erection products like Viagra and Cialis. These products were first developed to help heart patients and diabetics who could benefit from increased blood flow. However, during studies in heart patients, the biggest and most noticed side effect was huge and frequent erections. This side effect changed the nature of the product and spawned the multi-billion dollar market.

NO boosters have a cult following among bodybuilders who LOVE the pump associated with taking products. NO products seem to increase the pump associated with lifting, which can feel good and provide some benefit in recovery. There are many variations on the market and hundreds of products. Most will be a combination of the following products.

Arginine AKG

Arginine Alpha Keto Glutarate was the first big commercial NO product to hit the market. It seems to have some ergogenic benefits and seems to increase NO as well or better than other Arginine-based products. Alpha Keto Glutarate is a glutamine intermediate which should provide some decent recovery benefits. This product is a proven NO booster that seems to provide ergogenic benefits. These products can influence both growth hormone levels and recovery via multiple pathways. AKG has been shown to increase muscle levels of Arginine, so the combination is a good one.

L-Arginine

This is just the base amino acid. It seems to have some direct NO benefits over Arginine AKG since it is better at boosting vascular NO, where Arginine AKG seems better at boosting cellular arginine levels. The combination of L-Arginine and Arginine AKG seems to be the best way to boost NO via Arginine. L-Arginine is directly converted to NO and provides a much needed increase in vascular NO. That being said, it is often excluded from many NO products because it is viewed as cheaper than Arginine AKG.

Arginine Malate

This is L-Arginine bonded to Malic Acid. The theory behind this supplement is that Malates are intermediates in the Krebs cycle and is used to recharge the body's energy system. It comes in 2:1 and 1:1 ratios of Arginine to Malic Acid. The 2:1 seems to be the superior mix, but it is relatively unknown whether this is true. DiArginine Malate seems to be a good NO potentiator and has some very good anecdotal data behind it. Often, you will find this supplement mixed with other forms of Arginine.

Arginine Ethyl Ester
Here we go again with another useless form of amino acid. The ethyl ester craze has given us as many versions of aminos bound to ethyl esters as any other sports supplement. The problem is that they have never been proven to do anything above their amino acid counter parts and could potentially have a lesser effect in the body. They are reported to increase absorption by making the amino acids less polar and there for helping them though the gut, which is almost laughable. Again, I would stay away from this product unless you want to waste money. Recently, using creatine as a model, very little blood esterase (the enzyme that cleaves the "ester") acted on amino acid esters, making them very unlikely to be good candidates for esters.

Arginine Orotate
This is just simply L-Arginine bound to Orotic Acid. Orotic Acid has many ergogenic benefits, including being able to increase endurance. This should be a very good ingredient and has lots of solid scientific information behind it. Orotic Acid is one of the best chelating agents for minerals and has a lot of study information on it being part of an ergogenic enhancement compound.

Citrulline Malate

This amino acid (Citrulline) is an important metabolite of Arginine in the body and it is actually used by the cells to increase the amount of NO and Arginine. It seems to have a really good benefit when you add it to Arginine supplements and, on its own, is a proven endurance enhancement product. CM should be taken at 2-3g per day which is high for most supplements since they usually contain 1g of Cirulline Malate or less. At lesser doses, it doesn't seem to do much for endurance, but can certainly help recharge NO and Arginine levels. This is a very good ingredient and is useful in any NO boosting supplements. Citrulline Malate also buffers lactic acid, which makes it a great ingredient to add to Beta Alanine for muscle endurance.

Agents Added To NO Boosters

NorValine

This amino acid isomer has NO protective benefits that help NO hang around longer in the body. It is quite expensive and often used at levels that are too low to make a difference, but it is a very good supplement that can be used with any NO boosting agent to increase the "pump" effect.

Pomegranate

Pomegranate has been shown in multiple studies to protect the NO molecule and increase its life. This protective effect is why it is good to add to NO products. Pomegranate has a multitude of health benefits, but to NO products, it is a very good addition to make L-Arginine more effective.

Grape Seed Extract (GSE)
Similar to Pomegranate, the pro-antocyanadins in grape seed seem to protect vascular NO and increases its effects. GSE has been shown to strengthen blood vessels and increase their flexibility.

GABA
This supposedly helps open up blood vessels along with increasing NO. I have taken it and I have not seen much of an effect from it. However, I have spoken to many other people that swear by GABA for its NO benefits. It does have some good neuro relaxing effects though.

Jujube Fructus
This fruit extract has been also shown to protect NO from degradation and to increase its effects.

Topical Arginine
This is an amazing find, although most people don't believe it works. Topical Arginine and NO boosters have been well-studied in diabetics and have shown increased blood flow over the course of a week of supplementation with topical L-Arginine. The most amazing thing about this supplement seems to be the amazing restorative and pain management effects of topical Arginine. Topical Arginine can be used in sexual enhancing products as well. I can tell you from personal experience that it does indeed work for that effect. You can make your own topical Arginine by combining it with water and alcohol or buy one of the many interesting products on the market.

Glutamine – healing agent or worthless?

L-Glutamine is SWORN by all the old school bodybuilders to be the best recovery agent on the market. It is true that Glutamine is used up and used in recovery, but the question is whether any of it actually makes it to the muscle to be used in recovery and regeneration. Oral L-Glutamine is very good for you and it is metabolized in the gut by intestinal bacteria. It helps them grow and produce positive metabolites that give the intestines proper balance. Additionally, Glutamine is converted to sugars by the body, so it is not really evident that supplementing L-Glutamine does anything positive for the bodybuilder. Still, one can't dismiss the many positive reports of Glutamine supplementation. Research shows that after intensely working out, glutamine levels in the body are reduced by as much as 50%, which is the basis for its view as a recovery agent. It has also been given to burn victims to help in their recovery, which shows at least some absorption. Glutamine has been shown to increase growth hormone levels, so there is really mixed reporting on its effects and in combination with Creatine to help strength and power in trained athletes.

L-Glutamine
The free form amino acid has been shown to be used in the gut for fuel by the intestinal bacteria and is the usual choice for supplementation.

Glutamine Peptides
These are wheat glutens that are partially digested. I am not a big fan of these because so many people have a partial or full

allergy to wheat. Peptides can have better absorption than the straight amino acids, but peptides from wheat and other sources that are partially hydrolyzed are not as good as those formed from free form amino acids.

Glutamine Ethyl Ester
Again, this is the ethyl ester version of Glutamine, which has really no data to support its use and seems counterproductive to taking amino acid complexes. There is no real reason to take Glutamine Ethyl Ester and I would avoid it. Recently, using creatine as a model, very little blood esterase (the enzyme that cleaves the "ester" acted on amino acid esters, making them very unlikely to be good candidates for esters.

RANKING INDEX

L-Arginine	★★★★★★
Arginine AKG	★★★★★
Arginine Malate	★★★★★
Arginine Orotate	★★★★★
Citrulline Malate	★★★★★
Arginine Ethyl Ester	★★★
Glutamine	★★★★
Glutamine Peptides	★★★★
Glutamine Ethyl Ester	★★

pSARMs, Herbal Testosterone Boosters, Herbal Adaptogens...

What are SARMs and pSARMs?

SARM stands for selective androgen receptor modulator. They are hormone like molecules that act like androgens or "anabolic steroids" in certain tissues without having the androgenic side effects of testosterone. The bad side effects of testosterone are hair loss and prostate enlargement, which a SARM does not promote. SARMs are in development from many sources and the popular prohormone 19Nor-Androstenediol was just reported to have SARM-like effects in men. Some SARMS are in development already including ARYL-PROPIONAMIDE and something code-named JNJ-28330835. The problem with these is that they don't provide fully equal muscle stimulation to testosterone and its metabolites so they lack the potency to be used as proper muscle building agents in younger men. SARMs are improving in potency and some day we may see a commercially available SARM but, for now, they are not available to the public as androgen replacement therapy or androgen augmentation therapy. SARM technology provides the most benefit to older men that want the muscle building properties and bone density increase that one receives from testosterone, but don't want the side effects like prostate enlargement that can effect men over 50.

pSARMs are phyto-SARMS or plant based SARMs. pSARMs can come in a variety of plant based sources and constituents that act as phyto-androgens in certain tissues. Phyto-androgens are available in many different forms but they usually share a similar structure and function. Often, they are closely related to phyto-estrogens and often mis-categorized because both androgens and estrogens are anabolic in bone, yet previously only estrogens were thought to be anabolic in bone. Phyto-androgens are great because they give similar muscle building effects like testosterone yet seem to lack the prostate and hair loss stimulation effects of testosterone and pro-hormones. Included, is a list of some of the more popular phyto-androgens on the market and a list of some items that are being called SARM's yet lack the science to be called a SARM.

What are Herbal Testosterone Boosters?

There are many herbal products that can boost testicular androgen production. These have been marked by many years of re-introduction of the same tired old ingredients with a few superstars appearing from time to time. Tribulus has a mix bag of reviews and it is really not a known quantity. However, at high doses and standardized, it does seem to have some effect.

Do SARMS and pSARMs build muscle?

SARMs by their nature are meant to be anabolic in muscle tissue. So, yes, in theory they should be potent or reasonably potent builders of muscle. pSARMs can indeed build muscle but that depends mainly on the potency and dose of the pSARM. If too little of the pSARM is used, the subject will get a negative result. With some of the more potent pSARMs taken at high doses they can mimic some of the effects of anabolic steroids. The trick is finding the right dose that stimulates muscle without having negative side effects in other tissues.

pSARM Theory of Activity

Testosterone Structure

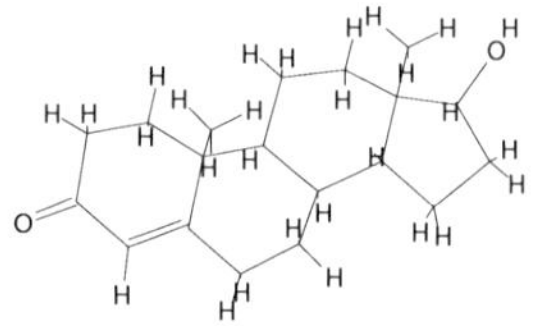

pSARM (Osthol)

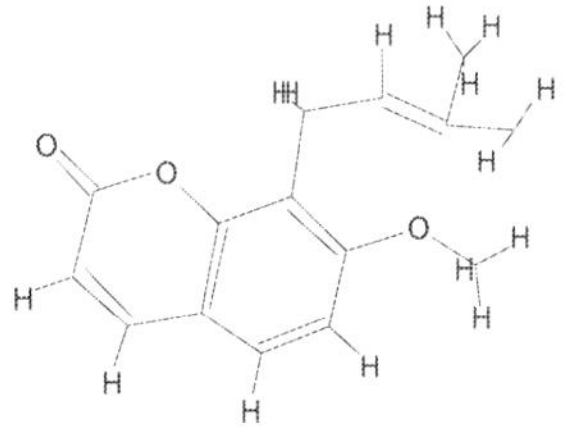

You can see how the two overlap and fit the binding pocket for the androgen receptor, which is why we believe the pSARM's to have their activity:

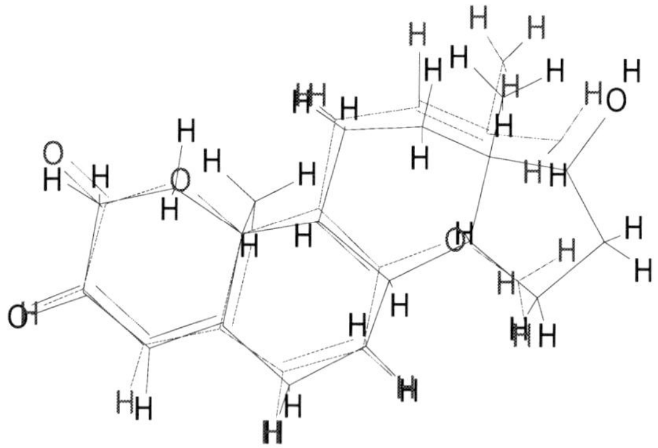

Icariin – the main phyto-androgen from Epimedium, or better known as Horny Goat Weed (HGW), has a study that shows it has phyto-androgen type effects. Although this paper isn't very conclusive and is quite weak on science, it is something of a start and HGW may have some anabolic effects. Unfortunately, real world results have not shown HGW to live up to the hype. However, it isn't a bad ingredient for other reasons (e.g., boosting NO and increasing sex drive). Some people speculate that HGW and its constituents have estrogenic effects, which wouldn't be a good thing, but Icariin doesn't seem to have that effect. So, look for HGW with a 70% or greater amount of Icariin. The verdict on this one is certainly not clear and it is too early to tell if this will make a solid pSARM. Icariin is something that might work, but the jury is still out on its usefulness.

Osthole (Osthol) – An extract of Cnidium, Osthole is shown in a few studies to have positive effects on NO and, in one study, to have phyto-androgen or pSARM activity. Also, this ingredient has been tested in many supplements and has a lot of anecdotal feedback on being effective. Look for at least an 80% extract to be potent enough to have a pSARM effect. Osthole seems to impart its effect by mimicking the effects of testosterone in specific tissues. This is probably one of the best phyto-SARMs on the market and real world results prove this to be a very capable pSARM that can have a positive effect on strength and endurance.

Hibiscus – This flower extract seems like an unlikely candidate for phyto-androgenic effects but it has been shown in many studies to have direct anabolic effects in muscle tissue. Hibiscus has been shown to be a potent stimulator of muscle growth and a sexual stimulant. Standardized Hibiscus extract is one of the most exciting finds to hit the market recently. The two major Hibiscus species that have anabolic properties are Hibiscus Rosa sinensis and Hibiscus Macranthus, both of which have been shown to have positive benefits. Stick to the water-based extracts since the ethanolic extraction method seems to pick up some negative ingredients that can cause issues.

Unknown Structure

White Ginger – Although this ingredient is tough to find, it does seem to have pSARM activity based on a few studies. White Ginger is not the same as the ginger we use for spices however. Straight ginger seems to have testosterone boosting effects while white ginger has direct androgenic effects, making it a potent pSARM. A supplement company that can find this extract stands to have a very popular and potent product.

Unknown Structure

Diandrone or Dianadrone – This is not a pSARM; it is simply the hormone DHEA. DHEA is not selective and is, indeed, an androgenic prohormone on its own. There is reason to use this in supplements, but it is not a pSARM at all, or a even a SARM for that matter. DHEA is a well-known hormone having slight androgenic activity on its own and can convert into testosterone. By itself, DHEA has been shown to not have any muscle building effect, most likely because of it being rapidly cleared from the body. However, this should not be classified as a pSARM.

Eucommia Ulmoides – This herbal ingredient seems to have a pSARM effect but is pretty hard to find in the standardization needed to elicit an anabolic effect. It has been shown that the constituents of Eucommia can have a direct androgenic effect on muscle and others (caprylates) can increase androgen sensitivity. It is certainly a very good candidate for a pSARM once a company figures out how to best standardize for its proper constituents. The raw bark would, theoretically, take grams to have a positive effect, making this impossible to use as a supplement.

Herbal Testosterone Boosters

These items are reported to boost testosterone, but are low on real scientific data. Many of them do boost sex drive, which is why they are reported to increase testosterone, but that isn't necessarily true. Sex drive can be increased through other mechanisms like with yohimbe, so don't take this effect as anything to necessarily do with testosterone. Still, it is possible to boost testosterone through these mechanisms.

Tribulus Terrestris- This ingredient is often over-used and reported as the "gold standard" in testosterone boosters. It has been shown in multiple human studies to not boost testosterone at all or affect androgen levels in general. It is thought to stimulate LH, although this is an unproven. It has been shown in many animal studies to have a positive effect on sex drive, but again in humans, it is proven to not work. Critics of the human studies will challenge the dose and standardization of the extracts studied. It is a decent ingredient for the price, but don't spend a fortune on it and look for blends with herbal extracts that are better suited for testosterone boosting effects.

Maca – Maca has shown to have no positive effect on testosterone, nor is it a valid pSARM. Maca most likely works by reducing the amount of estrogen and DHT in the system, which is useful but isn't a pSARM or phyto-androgen effect.

Fenugreek – Similar to ginger, this is a spice that has shown testosterone stimulating properties, but it does not have pSARM activity or any androgenic activity on its own. It is useful in testosterone boosting supplements, but lacks the direct effect. Still, Fenugreek can be a solid addition to any testosterone boosting supplement.

Tonkat Ali (Eurycoma Longifolia) – This herb has many studies showing it to be an adaptogen and herbal testosterone stimulant. Some people are trying high doses as a pSARM but the verdict is still out. Still, it is useful as a testosterone booster and adaptogen, so it is a good addition to a pSARM formula.

Bassella Alba – This is not a pSARM, but it does seem to have potent testosterone stimulating effects. Although not a pSARM, it is still useful in testosterone boosting supplements and has a very positive study showing it to boost testosterone. Although it is new, it is a pretty killer ingredient for a testosterone booster.

Avena Sativa - Wild Oat Straw doesn't seem to boost testosterone, but may inhibit SHBG, which can free up bound testosterone. It is best stacked with other herbal boosting supplements to increase their effect since SHBG is a main way that testosterone gets inactivated in the body.

Dodder Seed - Shown in several studies, Dodder Seed seems to be able to naturally boost testosterone by increasing LH. Dodder seed is pretty new but shows some promise in the testosterone boosting market.

Urtica Dioica – Better known as stinging nettle, this is probably the most versatile plant for a male or female looking to boost androgens. It contains extracts that reduce estrogen, reduce DHT and reduce SHBG. All of these things are really useful for the bodybuilder, both male and female. There is a recent trend to standardize for just 3,4-divanillyltetrahydrofuran but the raw herb in a 10:1 extract is a much better choice since nettle has so much to offer the bodybuilder.

Cordyceps sinensis – This fungus has been shown in Chinese studies to boost sexual activity and is also an adaptagen. It was also shown in rat studies to boost testosterone. It was brought to market with much fanfare, but it didn't seem to live up to the hype. Many people are reporting that up to 1200mg of Cordyceps is not having a positive effect on body composition or strength and endurance.

ZMA (R) – ZMA is composed of three/four nutrients that have some limited ability to increase the effect of testosterone. The nutrients are Zinc Asparate, Magnesium Asparate, Zinc Methionine and B6. In clinical trials, this combination has shown not to raise testosterone or provide any body composition benefits. There is one big benefit of Zinc however, which is to increase the sensitivity of the androgen receptor, which could make testosterone more active in some people.

This however can be achieved via Zinc supplementation alone and does not require high priced combinations to achieve its effect. The other two ingredients are just window dressing in my opinion since B6 can be gotten from food in and fortified foods and magnesium, while great for you requires higher doses to be effective. ZMA is not bad for you, it just doesn't warrant the high price that it commands.

Avena Sativa – Avena Sativa is simply oat straw or the part of the plant that they throw away when they are done harvesting oat meal. Avena Sativa does have a decent effect, which is to possibly increase free testosterone via SHBG bocking. As a first attempt SHBG blocker, it was innovative 10 years ago, but today many better products have replaced it as the premier SHBG blocker like Stinging Nettle Avena Sativa isn't necessarily a bad thing when taken as a supplement, it is just not that great of an ingredient for raising testosterone.

Tribulus Aquaticus – this ingredient has zero information substantiating it as a testosterone booster however it does have some anecdotal reports of people liking its effects. Still, without even one study showing this to do anything, it is probably one to watch for it's adaptogenic effect if nothing else.

Chlorophytum Borivilianum - This is a pretty neat herbal that has some decent science behind it showing it to be an aphrodisiac that increases sperm quality and quantity. These herbals don't usually show up as testosterone builders, but still make a fine part of an herbal testosterone/sexual aid.

Non-Hormonal Anabolics:

This list of ingredients have reported anabolic effects that do not rely on testosterone. They typically work in other pathways that are anabolic, yet not androgenic. There are many pathways that do have this effect like IGF-1, MTOR and further down stream metabolites. Research on these is still new and although these agents don't typically put the same amount of muscle on as hormonal items, they still have some great benefits!

Beta Ecdysterone -

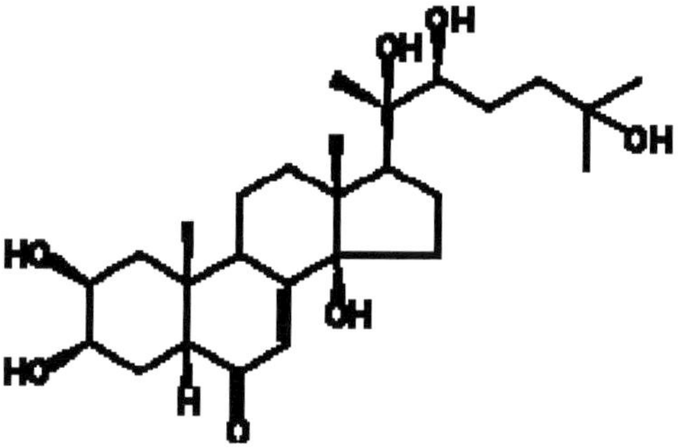

This is another ingredient that is constantly reconstituted in an effort to make it sound cool and anabolic. Some research was done in the 60's on ecdysterones having anabolic effects and then it basically went dark. There is some reason to suspect that these bug steroids do have activity in primates, but it is not really strong. Either way, it seems the rapid clearing of ecdysterones in the body make it impossible to make a very good oral product. I have personally tried over 1200mg per day of oral ecdysterone and it had no effect. I believe that the studies were done with injectable ecdysterones, which is why most commercial products don't work. The positive studies have shown in immature rats to rival Dianabol, but real world results have not proven this to be true as an oral agent. Ecdysterone can be modified to potentially increase the bioavailability by including things like esters and ethers, but up to this point no commercial product includes such modifications. Recent papers in mature mice show that it does increase strength and muscle weight, it must be just about the delivery method.

Diosgenin - This is an extract from Wild Yam that is converted in large fermentation vats to DHEA. Diosgenin has not shown to have any intrinsic anabolic activity nor can it be converted in the body to DHEA. This ingredient is pretty much a bust, as far as anabolic agents go, and would avoid it for the most part. It won't do any harm, but it won't do much good either. There is one study showing it to have anabolic effects in female rats, but that is sorta sketchy.

6-Keto-Diosgenin - There is really no evidence on this item either. This is a 6-Keto derivative of diosgenin and it is also reported in the Russian papers that it does have an anabolic effect. I have never used this but the reports do seem to be pretty good that it builds muscle and that it is anabolic.

20-Hydroxy-Ecdysterone – This is just another name for Beta Ecdysterone. There are many variants to the basic ecdysterone molecule that have about the same effect, making them pretty much interchangeable as a supplement.

Ecdysterone Acetate – This is simply an esterfied version of ecdysterone. This actually has some serious potential for prolonging half life by blocking enzyme clearing sites. The ecdysterone poly-acetate is the most likely form that we will see on the market.

Turkesterone –

This is another bug steroid that was shown to be even more potent that Beta Ecdysterone at building muscle. Unfortunately, this product probably has the same metabolic clearance issues as Beta Ecdysterone, but if you can find a good dose of full extract, it is worth a try. It is about 20% stronger than regular ecdysterone, but it usually only comes in very low doses because of the cost.

Cissus Quadrangularis – This ingredient was first brought out as a joint repair supplement and it seems to have a very positive effect on joint health. More recently, it was found to be a pretty potent cortisol blocker and insulin modulator. It has been shown to help with a variety of metabolic syndrome effects and anecdotally has some great feedback on its ability to build muscle.

5-Methyl-7-Methoxy-Isoflavone – Better known as methoxy-isoflavone, was the first product purported to be a pSARM since it was reported to be anabolic. Unfortunately, the real world results have not panned out in this case and methoxy isn't a very good oral ingredient. There is some support for it, topically, in a transdermal but these are hard to find. Every few years some company re-releases methoxy-isoflavone as a "wonder supplement", but it is certainly not very useful as an oral anabolic agent.

Ipraflavone – Similar to methoxy-isoflavone, this product is almost identical to the above Methoxy-Isoflavone in effect and criticism. Ipraflavone is not proven in real world tests to do anything anabolic in muscle. It is probably estrogenic and is used in many women's formulas to increase bone density.

Forskolin – This extract of the coleus forskohlii plant is supposed to have benefits that rival the illegal steroid Anavar. Real world examples are quite convincing that Forskolin has some very good benefits. It increases cAMP levels in the body, which can have profound effects on many bodily functions including: inhibition of platelet clumping; inhibition histamine release; increased force of contraction of heart muscles; relaxation of the arteries and other smooth muscles; increased insulin secretion; and increased thyroid function that shows it can readily affect multiple tissues. Additionally, it has been shown to upregulate 3bHSD. So, taken with Androsterones, it has a positive effect on hormonal conversion. It would seem that Forskolin has a very good chance at being a non-hormonal anabolic and is a good addition to a supplement or on its own.

Adaptogens:

These products help the body to "adapt" to stress and increase recovery and work output. They are not muscle building agents but they can go a long way to help you have a much better workout and reduce fatigue. They have history as herbal products that increase energy and, for the most part, they seem to live up to their reputation. Although not really critical in building muscle, these ingredients can go a long way in increasing overall ability to work out more often.

Ginseng – The first and most popular adaptogen, I don't really see ginseng as a useful ingredient for most males. It has been shown to have some estrogenic constituents and should probably be avoided. That being said, so many people like it for its mental stimulation effects, that I guess it should be considered as "under consideration" for bodybuilding purposes. It can help increase NO and thus helps with erectile issues, which is probably why it is classified as a sexual stimulant.

Bacopa Monniera – This is another herbal adaptogen that has been shown to increase memory and mental acuity. Unfortunately, it is a mild sedative, which makes it good for relaxing at night, but not really great to take before a workout because you want your senses at their height. Only take this if you have chronic stress or as a relaxing supplement at night. Otherwise, avoid items that have a sedative effect. One other interesting thing about Bacopa is that it increases the conversion of T4 to T3, making it a pretty good thyroid stimulator.

Rhodiola rosea – This is really the premier adaptogen since it has human clinical data showing it increases exercise performance. Performance doesn't exactly mean muscle growth but it does seem to help the bodybuilder recover from workouts faster and increase intensity while reducing fatigue. It would be best to have this on-hand to help you recover from grueling workouts or to use prior to a tough workout where you just "don't feel like it". According to the literature, rhodiola's effects seem to wear off after a couple of days, so it is best to use it only when needed.

Ashwagandha – This is another adaptogen that has positive effects on the neurological system. It has been shown to lower cortisol by up to 28% and increase feelings of restfulness, energy, sleep quality and well being. This herb has some positive benefits for the bodybuilder since reduced cortisol can certainly be a good thing in general and following a cycle of any hormone product. Of all the adaptogens this is probably the best for the bodybuilder!

Terminalia Chebula - This herb seems to have many positive effects. It has been shown to be an anti-inflammatory, antibiotic, anti-oxidant and helps with gastric clearing. By the profile this is probably an adaptogen, but there is not clear data showing it to have this effect.

RANKING INDEX

PSARMS:

Osthole	*****
Icariin (Horny Goat Weed)	****
Hibiscus	****
White Ginger	No Data
Dianadrone	Misclassified
Eucommia	No Data

Testosterone Boosters

Urtica Diocia	*****
Funugreek	*****
Tonkat Ali (Longjack)	*****
Bassella Alba	*****
Tribulus	****
Dodder Seed	****
Cordyceps	****
Avena Sativa	***
Macca	***
Zinc, Mag, B	**

Anti Estrogens? Do they build muscle?

The answer, if taken alone, is a resounding NO.. However, as part of a solid pyramid program, they can boost testosterone above levels seen in normal males. The average male has a testosterone level that is between 300 and 700 nano-grams per deca-liter of blood (ng/dl). This broad range is affected by a variety of factors and aromatase is one of them. Most AI's have shown the ability to raise testosterone to levels approaching 1200ng/dl but this ahas never translated into muscle growth. You may have heard the term PCT on many of the steroid forums. After a cycle of pro-hormones and steroids, the male testes tend to shrink and lower natural production and the use of anti-estrogens helps reverse this effect faster than natural recovery alone. With anti-estrogens, there are two basic technologies that have similar effects.

The first are anti-aromatase agents, which limit the aromatase enzyme that converts testosterone to estrogen. The body has a feedback mechanism for estrogen that senses when estrogen levels get too low (the male body DOES need estrogen to function). If the estrogen levels get too low, then the body responds by making more testosterone which in theory converts to estrogen and corrects the problem. Estrogen (or lack of) is sensed by the pituitary gland and the testes are instructed via Luteinizing hormone to make more or less testosterone. So, by lowering estrogen artificially, the body is told to make more via increasing testosterone.Anti-aromatase agents temporarily lower estrogen to trick the body into producing more testosterone. This actually works really well, but there can be negative effects. Prescription Anti-Aromatase products are Arimidex(R), Letrozol(R) and Exemestane(R). These ingredients are illegal to sell to males except for special circumstances like breast cancer, but we have many natural agents that do the same thing which is great for the bodybuilder who is trying to increase natural testosterone levels or recover from a cycle of steroids.

Conversion of Testosterone to Estradiol Via Aromatase:

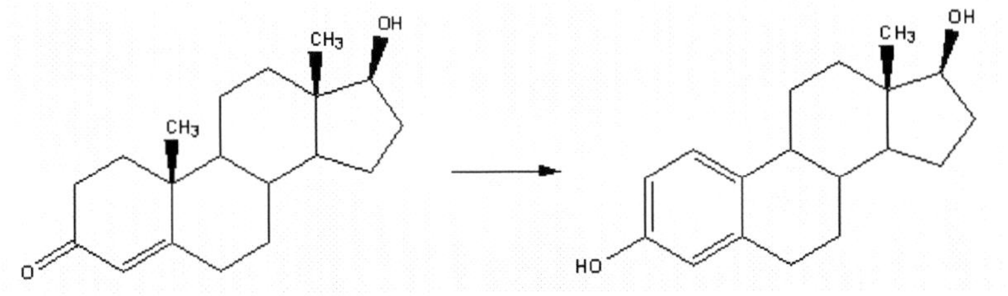

Conversion of Androstenedione to Estrone Via Aromatase:

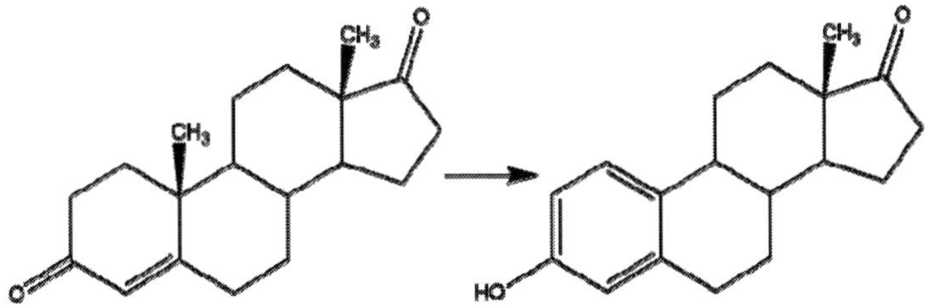

Aromatase Inhibitors:

These limit the conversion of testosterone to estrogen by binding and inactivating the aromatase enzyme, which has the downstream effect of raising testosterone via a feedback loop that is dependent on estrogen (estrogen is reduced, so the body creates more testosterone as a raw material) AI's have two methods of reduction. First, there is a suicide inhibitor, which locks up and deactivates the enzyme. The other method, competitive inhibition only temporarily blocks the enzyme from having activity. The items on the bodybuilding market are suicide inhibitors, which still work well enough to cause a major increase in testosterone for most males however these will not really work in females unless via some other pathway such as DHEA. Sadly in the current studies, this reduction in estrogen and the boost in testosterone doesn't translate into muscle gain, which is puzzling. I think if properly stacked with other items this could be a very good way to increase testosterone, but it seems that the body has many ways of reducing excess testosterone or the lab is seeing cross reaction which is the AI itself "looks" like testosterone on the test. The debate of whether to use AI's as a valid means to boost testosterone is one that is heated. Many experts and honestly most pharmaceutical steroid recovery agents are competitive ER inhibitors like Tamoxifen (NolvadexTM) which is interesting. The problem with any of the competitive receptor blockers on the market is that they suffer from rapid metabolic clearing via sulfation and glucoronidation.

This process is how the body removes anything that isn't food and there is a ton of it in the liver, making oral products very difficult design with any positive effect due to the rapid clearing of the ingredient. Ways around these metabolism routes are sublingual delivery (under the tongue), transdermal delivery (on the skin) or by blocking them with additional items that compete for the enzyme.

Chrysin

Chrysin was the first natural anti-aromatase or AI (aromatase inhibitor) on the market. Unfortunately, this ingredient never really panned out to much of anything. It doesn't seem to work in the body at all, which is odd since it works really well in the test tube. In the test tube, chrysin inhibited aromatase very well. However, it seems that once taken orally, or even injected, it is ineffective at doing anything. So, companies that are still using chrysin as their aromatase inhibitor are really wasting money and making ineffective supplements. I have some thoughts on why chrysin isn't effective, but I won't share those in case I ever want to release an effective chrysin supplement that works.

Androstene-3,6,17-trione

This ingredient was brought to market in 2002 as the next revolution in Aromatase Inhibitors. In fact, this steroidal AI does work and it works really well. It does exactly as advertised, increasing testosterone and reducing estrogen. There are some drawbacks with this ingredient but it is a very good AI and seems to improve testosterone levels to a good degree. The only downside to this ingredient is the need to take excessive amounts to see results and that the increased testosterone doesn't seem to result in more muscle. The recommendation is to take 600mg per day of this ingredient, making a $40 bottle good for only 10 days at this dose. It seems as though you can get away with 300mg and get about the same results though, and it is not uncommon for supplement companies to suggest that you take excessively high doses in order to get more money from you.

4-Hydroxy-Androstenedione – Formestane

This was the first steroidal anti-aromatase brought to market. It is actually a prescription drug in other countries. This product seems to lower estrogen without having as good of a testosterone boosting effect. This is pretty debatable, with evidence on both sides, so it looks like Formestane is a pretty potent AI that can be of benefit for the bodybuilder looking to control estrogen and increase androgenic effects and levels. High doses of Formestane can actually be a potent prohormone on its own, which is the basis for it being doubted to raise testosterone.

3-OHAT – 4-etiocholleve-6,17-one, 3b-ol propionate

This product is similar to the first item, the 3,6,17 dione, in that it is a 3b-ol variant of androstenetrione. It is a weaker AI, yet it seems to have a more potent effect when esterified and a lesser effect on its own. Similar to androstene-3,6,17-trione, it should be used similarly as well at doses of 200-400mg. Oddly enough, some companies promote that this is a pro-hormone, which is 100% untrue. Also, I have heard of some weird things like using this in a protein powder, which is an unusual thing to include. I would stay away from companies using these items in this way. It shows that they have no idea what they are doing. Still, there is a use for this stuff in place of other AI's and it should act in a similar capacity.

3b-Hydroxy-Urs-12-ene-28-oic acid

This is a new semi-steroidal aromatase inhibitor that has some real promise. It has other health benefits like being an insulin mimetic agent as well as being a moderately potent aromatase inhibitor. The only thing that makes this a tough choice right now is the need for a better delivery system for it to be effective. It is possible that a mix of glucoronidase inhibitors and sulftransferase inhibitors could make a big difference or perhaps sub-lingual delivery (under the tongue). The world forgot about sublingual delivery, but it does have some serious benefits for many items. This item should benefit quite well from a sublingual or using a combination of blocker technology to make it work effectively.

mATD - 17a Methyl 1,4,6 Androstatriene-3-one, 17b-ol

This is the 17aMethyl version of ATD. It could, in theory, have androgenic effects and we have no way of knowing if it actually reduces estrogen. This product can also cause liver stress and should probably be avoided until there is more research on this item. Most likely, it has some minor direct androgenic effect, which is why the companies selling it are trying to sneak it in as an anti-estrogen. The reality is that there are much better pro-hormones on the market if you want to really take an androgenic product. So, taking methyl-ATD isn't really worthwhile. There is also some confusion whether this product is a 4,6 diene or a 1,4,6 triene, which isn't a big deal since they have similar activity and function.

6-Bromo-Androstenedione

This is similar to many other steroidal anti-aromatase agents, and is on the market. It should be very good, but is in no way DSHEA compliant. It will reduce estrogen but could have secondary shut down via an androgenic pathway. Still, probably a decent AI with potent effects. There is a mix of 6a and 6b bromo groups on the market and some that have both. No one seems to understand which isomer is better. Until then, I would probably stick with something tried and true.

7,8 Benzoflavone

This new anti-aromatase is promised to be the strongest plant based AI on the market. Real world data has yet to be established, but this one does look very promising for anyone that can get it delivered properly. The only problem I see with this one is that Chrysin also looked great on paper and failed in humans when it was put to the test. Only time and a well documented study will prove this one for sure but it looks like a strong contender for plant based anti-aromatase agents. Unfortunately, just putting this in a pill without some serious bio-availability nutrients isn't going to cut it. If someone can get it to work, it has an even stronger ability to reduce estrogen than ATD.

Estrogen Blockers – Selective Estrogen Response Modifiers (SERMS)

Much like a football player needs to block to be effective, estrogen blockers get in front of the "real" estrogen in your body and stop its effects. This is done by binding the estrogen receptor and doing nothing or having a weak effect. Blocking raises testosterone because the body is unable to get the same effect from the estrogen blocker and thinks there is a shortage of estrogen then the body releases more LH to increase testosterone production. This has a positive effect of not changing the body's own estrogen levels, yet still increasing testosterone and is the preferred method of testosterone production. The major problem is that estrogen blockers were either sold in the underground grey market, such as tamoxifen (trade name Nolvadex) or clomiphene (Clomid), or ineffective. There are many natural estrogen blockers, both partial agonists (having a weak effect compared to estrogen) and antagonists (having no effect, yet still binding to the estrogen receptor), yet they all have problems with oral bio-availability. That is the trick, finding new ways to deliver natural phytoSERMS. They are there, but like the plant-based aromatase inhibitors, they need a better delivery system like sublingual or otherwise.

PHASE 3 — NATURAL SERM INTRODUCTION

NORMAL CELL | ESTROGEN BLOCKED CELL

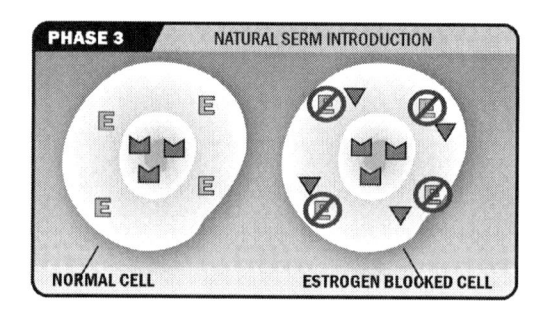

Resveratrol

First extracted from wine, resveratrol makes an excellent SERM type product that has many other health promoting benefits like anti-aging and cardiovascular. Resveratrol has been shown in studies to raise testosterone, block estrogen and increase LH. The major problem with Resveratrol is the delivery system. It is rapidly metabolized and excreted by the body, making it unlikely that oral doses ever get to have an anti-estrogen effect in the cells. A new sub-lingual resveratrol is on the market and promises to increase the absorption of this amazing nutrient and has benefits for anti-aging and estrogen blocking.

Ellagic Acid

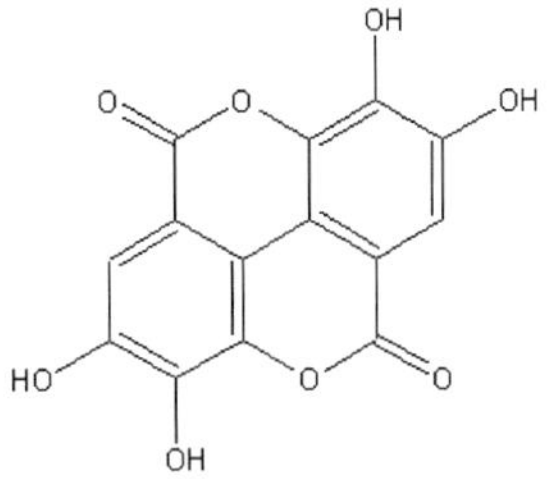

This extract of raspberries and pomegranate has true SERM-type effects. It has been studied to block estrogen, yet there is no data on it increasing testosterone. Still, this is the only ingredient available to mimic the powerful effects of true SERMS (most others are ERM's, meaning they are not selective). Ellagic Acid also has anti-cancer effects, along with a host of other health benefits. Ellagic Acid comes in many different strengths ranging from 40% (most common) to the highly potent 95% quality. It is commonly found in raspberries, but can also be found in including raspberries, strawberries, cranberries, walnuts, pecans, pomegranates and other plant foods.

Daidzein

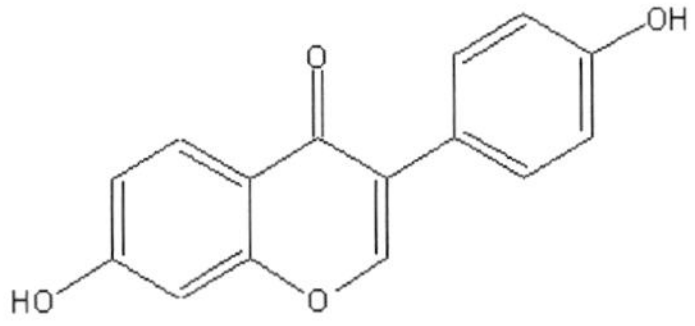

Daidzein is a metabolite of soy that has weak estrogenic activity. This is a classic partial agonist, meaning it has some estrogenic activity, but is nowhere near as potent as the estrogens in the body. This will have the effect of making the body increase LH while still having the benefits of estrogen in the body without being 100% devoid of estrogenic activity. This is good for both men and women.

Flavones

All of the flavones in sports supplements are usually rapidly metabolized and have a variety of effects. They have not shown over multiple products to be able to actually do anything to boost testosterone. These products have a variety of modifications. Hydroxy-Flavone and Methoxy-Flavone derivatives are on the market but they have not proven to be useful in real world examples.

Estrogen Clearing Agents:

These help detoxify estrogens in the body and clear estrogens more quickly. Unfortunately, these seem to have anti-androgen activities and reduce the anabolic/androgenic environment in the body. They would be good if you had gynecomastia symptoms along with something androgenic. If not, I wouldn't take them.

Diindolylmethane – This phytochemical is a natural component of cabbage, brussel spouts and broccoli. It converts estradiol to a less potent estrogen, which reduces the effect of it in the body. This can be quite useful in treating breast cancer but the concern is that DIM is an anti-androgenic agent as well, which is not good for men.

Indole-3-carbinol – this is similar to DIM yet seems to be less potent at clearing estradiol from the body. It shares many of the same good and bad points as DIM and shouldn't be used by the bodybuilder unless there is an issue with gynocomastia.

The Bottom Line

Estrogen control products have their uses but they don't seem to work really well on their own, which is why we put them towards the top of the supplement pyramid. In controlled studies, AI's have been proven to boost testosterone but that hasn't shown to actually build muscle, showing that the body needs typically more than the normal range of testosterone to boost muscle growth. Still, they have some really good uses and it is great to have such a variety of agents available over the counter. If you have just taken a cycle of pro-hormones or even real steroids, these products offer some really amazing benefits that can be used by the bodybuilder. I also think that stacked with the basics, these products can take you to a level of performance that is unrivaled in history. The problem is that moderately high levels of testosterone, alone, will not build solid muscle, which is why we need to cover all the bases first and then additional testosterone can be a huge benefit.

Product Ranking Charts

Anti-Aromatase:

Androst-3,6,17-trione	* * * * *
1,4,6-Androstatrienedione	* * * * *
4-Hydroxy-androstenedione	* * * * *
3-OHAT	* * * * *
6-Bromo-androstenedione	* * * * *
Androsterone	* * * * *
3b-urs-12-ene-28-oic-acid	* * * *
7,8 Benzoflavone	* * * *
mATD (methyl-1,4,6)	* *
Chrysin	*

SERM:

Resveratrol	* * * * *
Ellagic Acid	* * * * *
Daidzein	* * * *

Pro-Hormones The Top Of The Supplement Pyramid

Pro-hormones

Pro-hormones take things to another level entirely. There are many types of pro-hormones on the market but they all have one basic thing in common; they are meant to convert into an active steroid in the body and raise the androgenic profile above things like testosterone boosters and anti-estrogens. There are some potential downsides to these dietary supplements but, overall, they have been proven over the past 10 years to be safe and effective if used properly. First, no one under 21 should use pro-hormone products, second you should make sure you understand the requirements, including the need for proper post cycle support. Third, you should understand that there are potential down sides to pro-hormone use, including acne, hair loss, potential gynecomastia and other issues.

A standard PH cycle should last between four and six weeks. The products should be taken with a fatty meal to help absorption and things that you should look for in your formulations to help increase absorption are things like Luteolin and Piperine, which block some of the enzymes in the stomach. These products are best taken over the course of the day with meals or a fatty snack. After the cycle, it is best to use a natural testosterone booster or anti-estrogen to cancel out any reduction in natural production.

1-Androsterone (DSHEA Compliant Pro-Hormone) also known as 1-Androstene-3b-ol,17-one

This product is the ultimate in strength and mass pro-hormone on the market. It is a very potent precursor to 1-Testosterone, which is 200% more anabolic than testosterone. It doesn't mean it will build 2X more mass than testosterone, it simply means that you need very little active product to get an anabolic response which is great for an oral product. 1-Testosterone cannot turn into estrogen and should have a lesser chance of hair loss than other products on the market because of its structure. It is extremely potent at 300-600mg per day and users report 10-15lbs of muscle in a 4-6 week cycle. 1-Androsterone is the ultimate product for anyone wanting size and strength, but it is something that should be used with caution since it is so potent and certainly should never be used by anyone under 21. Side effects are generally mild, but it has been reported that some people suffer from lethargy (fatigue) when taking this product which is reported to be diminished when the product is stacked. Also, sex drive varies among different people with this compound (which is common), so some people report major sex drive increases while others have just the opposite effect. The point is that everyone is different and these effects just happen to some people, not all people. The lethargy and the hair loss are certainly possible though and it is best to know that going in. Often the most potent compounds have the worst side effects, but this one is a good balance. Look for 1-Androsterone to be something that will change the face of sports supplements for those that want to go the hard core route.

End Conversion Steroid: 1-Testosterone
Androgenic Value: 135 - 135% of testosterone (1.35 times as androgenic as testosterone)
Anabolic Value: 200 - 210% of testosterone (2 times as anabolic as testosterone)

19Nor-Androsterone (DSHEA Compliant) – Also Known By: Norandrostene-3b-ol,17-one

This product is a precursor to nandrolone or better known as "deca". Nandrolone is a very anabolic hormone that is easier on the hairline and prostate than anything on the market. It does have a potential to cause you to lose sex drive because of its low androgenicity, but it is also 125% as potent as testosterone milligram per milligram, which causes quite an anabolic effect. It is a really good stacking product because it has so many positive benefits. The cost of this item is really the biggest down side. You will need to run at least 300mg per day of this alone to see positive benefits. It can convert to estrogen, but at a pretty slow rate, so gyno shouldn't be an issue. You can possibly stack it with other agents and run lesser amounts and get a much better effect. The final big benefit for this product is the joint repairing effect. Nandrolone metabolites seem to be able to stimulate repair of the joints and tendons, which is great for the bodybuilder! This is a potent product with a lot of potential to show amazing muscle growth and is very anabolic, it is just quite costly.

Overall this is one of the hottest new PH's on the market and you should jump on it while it is still around.

End Conversion Steroid: Nandrolone (deca)
Androgenic Value: 39 - 39% of testosterone (.39 times as androgenic as testosterone)
Anabolic Value: 125 - 125% of testosterone (1.25 times as anabolic as testosterone)

5a-epiAndrosterone (DSHEA Compliant) –
Also Known By: epi-hydroxy-etioallocholan-17-one

This pro-hormone is a precursor to Stanolone, which, is a very androgenic hormone that can, in theory, cause some hair loss issues. Oddly enough, this hasn't played out in the real world and this product is quickly becoming the favorite for people looking to cut up and gain strength. It should skyrocket your sex drive and increase intensity in the gym, which will certainly make you feel like working out even harder. Overall, it is a good builder, but not a mass monster, so it is suitable to stack this with other anabolic prohormones or alone if you are looking to do a lean bulk or cut. You should dose this at 300-400mg per day for 4 to 6 week cycles. It is a very good product that has some serious potential to build mass, along with other agents, or as a cutter on its own. However, don't look at it as the mass monster prohormone for your stack. The side effects seem very mild. Perhaps, one could get some acne and hairloss but it is not at all estrogenic and cannot convert to estrogen, making it safe for many different uses. Actively, it is about 2X as potent as testosterone in all tissues once you swamp the enzyme and get past the 3aHSD issue in skeletal muscle. Finally, this PH has some serious neuro-stimulating effects which can make your sex drive go through the roof.

End Conversion Steroid: Stanalone
Androgenic Value: 194 - 194% of testosterone (1.94 times as androgenic as testosterone)
Anabolic Value: 194 - 194% of testosterone (1.94 times as anabolic as testosterone)

11-keto-Androstenedione (DSHEA Compliant) – Also Known By: Adrenosterone

This is a prohormone found in fish. It is their primary hormone but is a metabolite of testosterone in humans. It is not a really potent pro-hormone but it certainly has some uses. Unfortunately, it will need to be taken at high doses to be an effective prohormone and even at that it isn't a really potent product. It does, however, reduce cortisol, which is great for getting lean. It is a good, stackable, product and gives great results when taken with other items. In theory, it can convert to estrogen but it would be a very weak metabolite that should have no estrogenic effects. Hair loss is in the same boat, so this makes it one of the safest PH's on the market. That safety comes at the expense of potency though and it isn't a really good product for those looking to maximize a cycle, but is a good product to stack with other items if you have some extra cash laying around.

End Conversion Steroid: 11-Keto-Testosterone
Androgenic/Anabolic Value: Unknown

Epi-hydroxy-etiochol-5-ene-17-one Ester (DSHEA Compliant)

This is a precursor to testosterone and other prohormones, it has good fat loss and anabolic potential. As a precursor to testosterone, it is a good base product to use for those that want to get started with pro-hormones. Testosterone is natural to the body, so it is probably the easiest product to get acclimated to and, if matched with the proper support nutrients, it can be the most potent product of the bunch. Since it is testosterone-based, it can convert to estrogen. So, look for something that controls estrogen in the formula. This will make the product stronger in addition to making it safer. It can convert to DHT, so look for something like stinging nettle or beta sitosterol to help stop this conversion, this will again increase the potency and increase the safety. If you are looking for a good base to any stack or a product to run as a first PH cycle, you can't go wrong with this product, just make sure your product has the proper support nutrients in there to make it effective.

End Conversion Steroid: Testosterone
Androgenic Value: 100 - 100% of testosterone
Anabolic Value: 100 - 100% of testosterone

1,4 Androstadiene-sterone
(DSHEA Compliant)

This product coverts to the steroid boldenone in the body. Boldenone isn't a particularly strong androgen, but it does have some things that make it good for a stacking item. 1,4 Andro can convert to estrogen, but it seems to do so at a slower rate than other items. It should also have a reduced effect on the hairline, so it is a pretty safe product in general. It is a decent stacker since it increases appetite and should help with endurance. It can also have a joint repairing effect, which is a good side effect. I have never heard of anyone gaining serious mass from Androstadienedione, even at 600mg per day, but it is a decent product for stacking. As you can see, it is also pretty safe, being about half as androgenic as testosterone with all of the anabolic effects.

End Conversion Steroid: Boldenone
Androgenic Value: 54 - 54% of testosterone (.54 times as androgenic as testosterone)
Anabolic Value: 100 - 100% of testosterone (As anabolic as testosterone)

4-Hydroxy-Androstenedione – Formestane

You might recognize this from the "anti-aromatase" section and indeed this product can do double duty (which is actually more common than you think). Given at semi-low doses this is a great anti-aromatase and testosterone booster but given at much higher doses (400mg+ per day) this makes for a prohormone to the steroid hydroxy-testosterone. Hydroxy-Testosterone is a potent steroid in its own right, not quite as anabolic as testosterone, but still quite potent. Many people were taking straight OHT (hydroxy-testosterone) before it was banned in 2004, so we know that OHT can be anabolic. It is about 75% as anabolic as testosterone, but don't let that fool you, at high doses Formestane is still a potent prohormone.

End Conversion Steroid: Hydroxy-Testosterone
Androgenic Value: 28 - 28% of testosterone (.28 times as androgenic as testosterone)
Anabolic Value: - 66% of testosterone (.66% as anabolic as testosterone)

Prohormones are really at the top of the food chain when it comes to mass building agents. They offer the best way to squeeze every ounce of extra muscle out of your workouts. Even though they are generally safe, they should be used with caution and under the supervision of a doctor. You should always discontinue their use if there is any issue that is uncomfortable or unusual. Pro-hormones certainly are nothing to play with, but if used properly, they are safe and effective with little chance for downsides.

Product Ranking Chart

Prohormones:

1-Androsterone	******
19Nor-Androsterone	*****
5a-EpiAndrosterone	*****
1,4 Androstadienedione	****
Epi-Hydroxy-Etiochol-5-ene	****
11-keto-Androstenedione	****

Sample Stacks:

Ultimate Mass Stack
1-Androsterone + Epi-HydroxyEtiochol-5-ene-17-one = Combination of wet and dry compounds for maximum gains

Dosage recommendation:
300mg 1-Androsterone +
340mg Epi-HydroxyEtiochol-5ene-17-one

Ultimate Wet Size Stack
19Nor-Androsterone + 1,4 Andro-dione = both can help you retain water weight for hard gainers who need instant "size"**Dosing recommendation:**
240mg 19Nor +
300mg 1,4 Andro

Ultimate Cutting Stack
5aEpiAndrosterone + 11-keto-Androstenedione = combination of anti-estrogenic, lipolytic and cortisol reducing effects
Dosing recommendation:
300mg 5aEpiAndrosterone +
300mg 11-keto-Androstenedione

Ultimate Safety Stack
19NorAndrosterone + 11-Keto-Androstenedione = combination of mild prohormones that should yield good effects.

**Dosing recommendation:
240mg 19NorAndrosterone +
300mg 11-Keto-Androstenedione**

Ultimate Strength Stack
1-Androsterone + 5aEpiAndrosterone = crazy strength gains (use the 5aEpi right before working out)
**Dosing recommendation:
300mg 1-Androsterone +
300mg 5aEpiAndrosterone**

Things added to Pro-Hormones

There are many things added to prohormones to make them more effective and less harmful. These items do a variety of things from limiting estrogen conversion to increasing absorption to modifying enzymes. Things like Stinging Nettle, Beta Sitosterol and others work on stopping the 5aReductase enzyme, making the conversion to 5aReduced versions lessened which can make the products more potent and reduce hairline issues. Second anti-estrogens can be added to block the aromatase enzyme or block inherent estrogenic activity like any of the above mentioned compounds like ATD as an AI or Ellagic Acid as a SERM. Finally, things can be added to increase the conversion quotient like Forskolin, which can upregulate 3bHSD and convert more of the prohormone to an active product. These are all good things if the company knows how to manipulate the chemical processes that are involved in conversion to active steroids and paves the way for a whole new process of increasing potency.

New Compounds on the horizon:

These compounds are new on the horizon and have some serious potential. I will only list compounds that have a chance of being DSHEA compliant and can be potent androgens on their own. These are not in production yet, but do have the ability to be on the market in the coming months or years. I strongly suggest any company do complete DSHEA studies on any of the androgens mentioned in this section to ensure legality in the US. These androgens are presented as fun information and as speculation on possible naturally occurring products in the food supply. This has not been verified yet via scientific study.

1,5 Androsterone - 3β-Hydroxy-1,5-androstadien-17-one

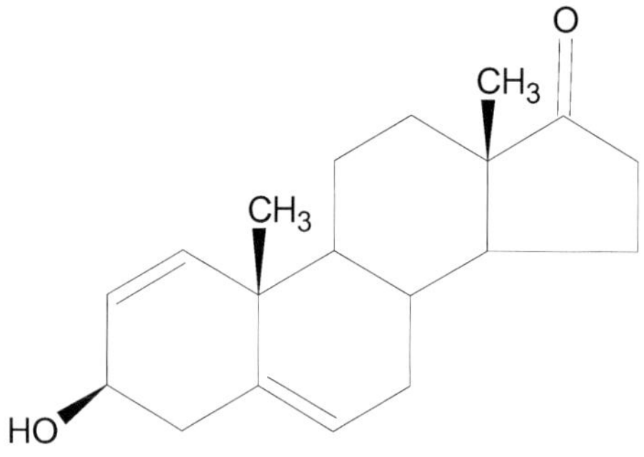

This product should be similar in strength to 1-Androsterone, yet have some of the possibilities of the 1,4 andro series. It is really an intermediate product that should, in theory, convert to

Boldenone and potentially further downstream a 1-Test analog. This one is too new to call, but the structure looks interesting. It is most certainly naturally occurring, probably found in a variety of pork tissues and potentially humans. It is one that probably won't see the light of day though, since it is an odd configuration and probably hard to make. The dione version might be interesting and more readily available.

Androgenic Value: Unknown
Anabolic Value: Unknown

estra-5(10)-ene-17-beta-ol – NorPentabol (tm)

This structure has some very good numbers on paper. It lacks the C-19 structure of testosterone, making it a nandrolone derivative, so it shouldn't really be able to convert to estrogen and it can't convert to any DHT type derivatives either. So, hairline shouldn't be a big concern with this one. It is a very unique structure with a potential to be a really good oral compound. It is very anabolic and seems to have a very good oral bioavailability, since the standard it is compared to is 17aMethyl Testosterone.

Androgenic Value: Unknown
Anabolic Value: 120 - 120% of Methyl-Testosterone (120% orally as anabolic as methyl-testosterone)

2,4-Dienedrol (tm) – 17-beta-hydroxy-androstan-2,4-diene

This structure is a modification of the popular Pheromone product on the market today. It seems to have a similar effect and structure to this pheromone, so it should have decent anabolic value. One difference is that this compound has the ability to most likely convert to estrogen, which isn't always a bad thing. It can also be a parent to the 2-ene pheromone via 5aReductase, so it should have some similar effects. This one is also about 120% as potent as testosterone, making it a pretty damn strong androgen and very low androgenic activity makes it a pretty good candidate for an oral androgen.

Androgenic Value: 40 - 40% of Testosterone (40% as androgenic as testosterone)
Anabolic Value: 120 - 120% of Testosterone (120% as anabolic as testosterone)

Fouronelone - 17-beta-hydroxy-5-alpha androst-2-en-4-one

Now we get to some really cool looking structures that are quite different from anything seen before in the steroid world. This structure has some serious potential to do a whole host of things. First, it is a pheromone derivative like many, but also has a 4-keto group, which should impart some possible anti-estrogen effects. This one can't really convert to much of anything, since the 4-keto will block both aromatase and 5a-reductase activity. When you look at the ratio though, it becomes apparent that this one has some serious potential for an active anabolic monster. It is 200% more anabolic than testosterone yet seems to have little androgenic activity from what I can gather. It should be pretty easily absorbed orally if you can protect the 17bHydroxy, so that should be a benefit as well.

Androgenic Value: ~25 - 25% of Testosterone (25% as androgenic as testosterone)
Anabolic Value: 200 - 200% of Testosterone (200% as anabolic as testosterone)

Gammadienedrol - 17-beta-hydroxy-5-alpha androst-1,3-diene

This one is another similar structure, having now a 1,3 diene, which should cause it to, again, be pretty inert to the standard estrogen converting and DHT converting enzymes. This one is fairly mild in comparison to other androgens in this section, but it is still pretty interesting for a potentially naturally occurring compound.

Androgenic Value: ~25 - 25% of Testosterone (25% as androgenic as testosterone)
Anabolic Value: 100 - 100% of Testosterone (100% as anabolic as testosterone)

Stimulants, GH Boosters and Unique Products...

Stimulants – They Build Intensity, Not Muscle

With ephedrine pulled off the market, there has been a rash of new products that are supposed to be "replacements" and better than ephedrine for burning fat. There are not many choices for fat burners on the market and even less that have a hope of DSHEA compliance. There are some that are reported to be DSHEA compliant but that is not 100% proven. Either way, it is possible that these ingredients are good when combined, but the reality is, nothing is as potent as ephedrine for stimulation and burning fat on a mg per mg basis.

Stimulants are really meant as intensity increasing nutrients. The only stimulant type product that has ever been shown to build muscle is the prescription product Clenbuterol. Unfortunately Clen causes heart damage and is pretty unsafe in general. Again, it won't kill you, but it is not anything to play with if you are seeking to stay healthy. Luckily, the right combination of nutrients can give you clen-like effects if you use them properly.

Caffeine

Caffeine

There is nothing in sports supplements that compares to adding caffeine to EVERYTHING. It is cheap and gives you a boost, which is why most companies add it to just about everything. Caffeine will get you going for sure, but it is not necessary to take massive amounts of caffeine from multiple sources. Everything from creatine to anabolics contain caffeine now, so it is pretty easy to get over 1200mg of caffeine per day for the average bodybuilder. Caffeine does have fat burning effects if you keep it in moderation. It is not bad to have some caffeine with your fat loss products, but it is best to get that from coffee since it can also help increase insulin sensitivity to counter act the caffeine effect. Caffeine overload and negative symptoms like insulin resistance can happen if too much is consumed.

Synephrine – Citrus Aurantium

The Bitter Orange can be standardized for synephrine, which is a stimulant in the ephedrine family, with lesser effects. Synephrine can actually help you lose weight, but it is not a real strong effect. Real world results show that this is not a replacement for ephedrine. However, it is useful in combination with other ingredients. Look for a supplement with synephrine for both the neuro-stimulation and the additional fat burning effects. There are some additional items that can help make a product stronger and reduce the metabolic clearing. Synephrine can certainly benefit from these additional ingredients. As a primary fat burner, synephrine isn't that good but, in combination, it is very useful. Recently, Methyl-Synephrine has hit the market and is being touted as the next coming. I have taken a few of these methyl-synephrine products and they didn't seem anything special to me. Modifications of this type are a shot in the dark, who knows if they work well or not. I would suspect that it is about the same as regular synephrine.

Yohimbine

The bark of the Yohimbe plant can be extracted for a compound called Yohimbine, which is a fat burning neurostimulant. It has blood flow increasing properties and targets stubborn body fat. It can even be used topically to treat tough areas. Yohimbine has only one serious downside; it can cause severe anxiety in some people even at very low doses. Hell, even for me the 6% extract makes me break out in cold sweats and extremely anxious. Oddly, the straight Yohimbine extracts (98%) does not have this effect. Even though people freak out with Yohimbe from time to time, it has been shown to be very safe. It was even tested as high as 30mg per day on men to treat erectile dysfunction, so the 3-5mg in diet products are certainly safe. It is great stuff when stacked with other stimulants because it works in other pathways besides the traditional routes.

Geranamine (TM) - 2-amino-4-methylhexane

```
      CH₃      CH₃
       |        |
       CH       CH
      /  \    /   \
    CH₂   CH₂      NH₂
    |
    CH₃
```

This is supposedly extracted from Geranium Oil, which makes it quasi-legal. It still needs some justification on this ingredient to make it 100% DSHEA compliant, but it is a pretty good ingredient and does seem to provide stimulation. It doesn't look like a potent fat burner but, when stacked with other items, it should do pretty well at increasing thermogenesis. I would suggest that this item really needs some support ingredients to help prevent it from being metabolized so quickly. All of these are good products for increasing intensity prior to working out and this one is certainly a good product for increasing both. On its own, it is not super potent, but it can certainly be stacked for maximum effect.

bPEA – Phenyl Ethylamine

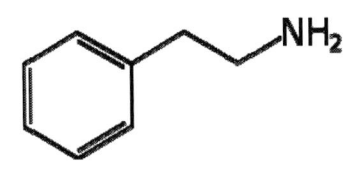

This is the stuff in chocolate that supposedly makes you feel good. It is a mood-enhancing product and doesn't seem to have much effect in the way of fat burning. That being said, feeling good and positive in the gym can be a really good thing! Unfortunately, this compound is rapidly metabolized by the body and excreted, so it is pretty tough to get an effective dose. It is often combined with MAO inhibitors. MAO is an enzyme that breaks down things like this and has a direct effect on dopamine. Some of the things PEA is stacked with include the herbs: Cat's Claw, Hordinine, Quercetin, Piperine and a few others. These don't seem to work very well so some people have tried to modify the PEA molecule. I have taken a few of these modified products and I have yet to notice anything significant from them. Still, stacked bPEA makes a good inclusion to a stimulant or diet pill.

Tyrosine

This amino acid can increase levels of dopamine in the body and also potentially increase thyroid output. T3 is 3 molecules of iodine bonded to one molecule of tyrosine. It also has dopamine stimulating effects and can increase focus and intensity. The N-Acetyl-Tyrosine seems to work much better than straight L-Tyrosine, but both will get the job done.

Theobromine

This is another coffee/chocolate extract that is very similar to caffeine in structure and function. It seems to have a slower and lesser effect compared to caffeine, meaning it lasts longer but doesn't give you much stimulation. Theobromine is a decent ingredient for increasing intensity, but its fat burning effect doesn't seem very significant. It is certainly a good support ingredient though and can help increase the effect of caffeine.

Guarana

This is just an herbal version of caffeine that is actually slightly different in how it is metabolized. It is broken down more slowly and hits you over hours vs. caffeine, which has a much faster effect. This makes guarana pretty good as an addition to a fat burner to help increase the effect. This wraps up a quick run-down of the stimulants. There are many other fat burning nutrients on the market and they are certainly too numerous to include in this book. Nothing I have found works incredibly well, except for Fucoxanthin. It seems to burn fat without a stimulant effect. That makes it a good (but expensive) addition to a supplement program. It is hard to gain muscle and lose weight, especially for you hard gainers who need to eat a ton just to put on any muscle, but it is possible with the right combination of nutrients.

Ephedrine

This of course was pulled from the American market officially in 2006. It is a very potent fat burner and has very good stimulating effects. It has been the subject of numerous studies showing it to be both safe and effective. Unfortunately, it had one minor problem, it can easily be turned into meth-amphetamines (crystal meth), which is why it was labeled public enemy #1 by the U.S. government. Don't believe that it caused that baseball player's death or any such craziness. Millions of ephedra and ephedrine pills were sold in the U.S. with no deaths or serious injuries. More people die of bee stings every year or coconuts falling then from Ephedrine, yet millions of people now live in complete fear of ephedrine due to propaganda.

Ephedra Leaves

Don't be fooled, this is all you will find on today's market that isn't a OTC drug. The bad news is that these new crop of ephedra leaves products don't contain any ephedrine (which is what made you lose the weight). This is basically a scam to get people to think that they are buying ephedra, but really buying the brown powder that is left after the ephedrine alkaloids are removed.

Methyl Synephrine

This is basically a structural modification to synephrine that seems to be more potent at burning fat. It is an ingredient that is short on information, but in theory looks interesting. I would say that this is probably pretty good, just lacks any clinical studies on what it does. Still, from the structure of the molecule we can predict it to be somewhere between synephrine and ephedrine in potency. It takes the basic Synephrine molecule and replaces the top hydroxyl with a methyl group, making it a hybrid synephrine/ephedrine molecule. Very interesting indeed, but certainly not 100% tested.

Octopamine

This is a chemical cousin to synephrine and ephedrine, but it is really meant for insects. It is their neurotransmitter and is a stimulant in their brains. This is probably why you find Octopamine in many plants. It's ability to stimulate mammals and people is questionable since seems to be rapidly cleared from the body. It is thought that it stimulates brown fat to help increase thermogenesis, but this was found to only occur in rats which isn't quite the same as in humans. Octopamine is a beta3-adrenoceptor agonist, meaning it stimulates that receptor subtype, however this receptor subtype doesn't seem to impart any neuro-stimulation effects. It's one to watch, but not 100% sure it is effective as a fat loss agent or stimulant.

Common Adrenergics

GH Products...prepare for the long haul

Growth hormone isn't the miracle muscle builder that is touted in these sports doping articles. GH, however, does have a place for those people that want to increase recovery, increase sleep related anabolism and increase satellite cells. The best growth hormone supplements can't even compare to injectable growth hormone, which takes 2-6 months to show any positive benefits. So, I think most people go into GH supplementation with the wrong attitude. GH supplements are for the elite athlete or older athlete that wishes to use these supplements for long term benefits.

Growth hormone is second only to Androgens in reshaping the body. GH has been proven to increase fat to lean mass ratio. In adult women, Growth Hormone caused a 4.6 lb fat loss with an increase of 6.6lbs of muscle. This is really the only "supplemental" agent to have such a profound effect.

Growth Hormone can be increased a variety of ways. First, it can be increased by blocking Somatostatin, which reduces and regulates growth hormone. This pathway is effected by most of your amino acids, they are wrongly called Secretagogues, but in fact they only block the negative feedback which tells your body to stop producing GH.

Second, the body can be stimulated to produce more of its own Growth Hormone Releasing Hormone via L-Dopa or something similar. This only works for a short time as your body becomes aware of the additional GHRH and reduces it other ways. This can be prolonged with the somatostatin blockers, but not indefinitely.

Third, the GHRH (growth hormone releasing hormone) receptor can be stimulated directly to increase production of GH in the pituitary. This is a very effective method of increasing natural GH production and represents the latest research in growth hormone releasing agents. There is no data on how long this can be done, but it seems like a much more effective way to increase GH long term and should probably be combined with the somatastatin blocking aminos to prolng life even further.

Finally, there is a third pathway, which utilizes Ghrelin (GHRP) to increase growth hormone release and this is not very well understood but seems to work in combination of GHRH release and actual stimulation of another receptor.

Arginine – This amino acid has been proven to release growth hormone in exercise trained men, which means that chronic use has some very good data behind it to show GH releasing properties.

Glutamine – This has also been shown in studies to increase growth hormone release in exercise-trained individuals and makes a very good amino acid to add to any GH releasing supplement.

Lysine – This amino acid has been shown to potentiate the effects of the other amino acids for GH release.

Arginine Pyroglutamate – Arginine has already been shown to increase growth hormone as does Glutamine and this supplement combines both into one peptide. This is simply Arginine bound to a cyclic glutamine peptide and it has been shown to have a better effect on GH than either arginine or glutamine alone.

Ornithine AKG - University studies have shown that Ornithine increases both insulin and growth hormone levels, which are needed to build and maintain muscle during intensive physical training. So, Ornithine has some serious beneficial effects for the bodybuilder. As the body ages, Ornithine may also help combat the muscle loss that is a normal part of the aging process. By helping to elevate growth hormone levels, Ornithine may help speed the production of muscle tissue and offset the effects of aging, which is of obvious benefit to the bodybuilder.

L-Dopa – This ingredient is the precursor to dopamine and has been shown to have a powerful effect on GH release it is extracted typically from Mucuna which contains a high amount of L-Dopa. It is also called "1C-Decarboxylase(TM)" in some supplements. L-Dopa can be used at high doses to treat Parkinsons, so it is quite safe at levels used in supplements. The best way to use L-Dopa is to alternate it every other week to make sure your body doesn't develop a tolerance to it. Still, it can safely be used every day to increase GH release, but it most likely will lose effect over time.

GHRP-2, Ghrelin – These are growth hormone releasing peptides that have some great short term effects when used as injectable products, but may be orally active on their own.

They show up in a few supplements, even though the synthetics are not 100% DSHEA compliant. Still, for someone with unlimited money to spend on GH supplements, GHRP-6 and GHRP-2 have some serious benefits when combined with the above supporting nutrients for GH release. They are best used on a 5 days on and two days off regimen. This represents one of the most effective GH releasing pathways available. Once someone figures out how to deliver it properly and can make it legal to sell in the US.

L-Tryptophan – This amino acid is back on sale in the U.S., thankfully, because it makes for one heck of a GH releasing product. Unfortunately, doses of 3-5g are necessary to achieve a positive GH response, making it a killer product to stack, but impossible to take in a combination supplement.

Astragalus – This herb has been shown, in a few studies, to release GH in rats, which makes it a decent inclusion. It is also a very good immune system booster and adaptagen, making it a good supplement for GH release.

Dioscitine – This ingredient is possibly one of the best growth hormone releasing agents to be discovered. It was shown in the scientific literature to increase GH production by over 17,000% (17.7 times greater growth hormone release) It does this by acting on the growth hormone releasing receptor, which is a separate receptor that releases growth hormone. This has yet to be tried in humans and real world data over time is not available but it looks very promising!

Puerariitine – This novel extract has the ability to increase growth hormone release via the GHRS receptor by over 170% (1.7 times baseline). This in combination with other GHRH releasing agents could make for an interesting product.

Dolichos Pruiens – this is simply renamed Mucunna pruiens or "L-Dopa" extract as mentioned above.

Other Interesting Products...

These items don't fit into any particular category but still have some neat benefits for the body builder.

6-Methyluracil - This product is one that has been shown to increase recovery in burn patients. It is an anti-catabolic agent that should help speed recovery in most cases. There is limited anecdotal support for this nutrient, but it is something that can be bought for recovery and ROS reduction.

Sodium Caprylate – This ingredient seems to have the effect of increasing androgenic activity at the receptor level. It has the potential to increase androgenic binding effects up to 250%, which makes it useful for anyone wanting to increase their testosterone booster, prohormone or even steroids. This ingredient is set to become something mainstream in its use to increase androgenic activity. However, it should be combined with a natural SERM in my opinion to reduce the chance of any estrogenic effects.

Astaxanthin – This ingredient is used in fish to provide that nice red color (salmon) and is a caratenoid from seaweed. This has some studies showing it to have an anti-catabolic effect in muscle, making it a recovery agent. It is pretty new and doesn't have much anecdotal information, so the jury is still out on this item.

Cystoseira canariensis – This ingredient was a supposed Myostatin blocker and was proven to not work at all. I would avoid this one.

Humanovar(tm) – This is an extract of chicken eggs that supposedly has steroid stimulant properties. This one has been around for a while but has been shown anecdotally to not really do much of anything. There are some rumors of a new version that is extracted for myostatin reducing properties, but that is all theory for right now. It is still around in a few supplements though on the shelves.

Gamma Oryzanol – This oil extract is reported to have testosterone enhancing effects. It was shown in a scientific study to have zero effect on testosterone or hormone levels, in general, but some people still swear by it. Maybe an adaptogen?

Dermatan Sulfate – This ingredient has been shown to increase mechano growth factor, which is a powerful signal for muscle growth. This, coupled with IGF-1, have the most potential in increasing genetic muscle growth. These items actually change the make-up at a cellular level.

Arachadonic Acid – This is a fatty acid that increases muscle damage and therefore sends a growth signal to the muscle cells to increase anabolism. It has been reported to increase weight loss and NO and is certainly a supplement to watch for future information. It has been shown to not impact muscle growth in trained men, but again with the proper support nutrients, it could be a good ingredient. The only issue with AA supplementation is that it can cause arterial damage, increased risk for stroke and cancer progression if used long term.

Phosphatidylserine (PS)- PS is a phospholipid that is derived from soy beans. PS has been shown to help control cortisol levels. Roughly 800 mg after training saves muscles by blunting the total amount of cortisol released by your body. This is good for short burst, since you do need cortisol for life and chronic suppression of cortisol can cause cortisol rebound. Another benefit is that when you keep cortisol levels under control, it's easier for your muscles to hold carbs.

Guggulsterones E&Z (natural or synthetic) – These potential fat burners have the ability to potentially ramp up T3 production. Unfortunately there is only limited information on this as an effect. Guggul has other important benefits like lowering cholesterol, making it pretty good for people who have cholesterol issues. Unfortunately, Guggulsterones have been shown to lower the effect of testosterone by acting as an androgen antagonist (blocking testosterone at the receptor). This makes them unpopular for most bodybuilders. Even the T3 boosting benefits of Guggulsterones probably wear off in two to three weeks as you body changes its production to buffer the increased effect.

7-Keto-DHEA (also 7-Hydroxy-DHEA) – 7-Keto-DHEA is a metabolite of DHEA that has no androgenic effects, meaning it will not build muscle via the androgen receptor. This being said, it does reduce cortisol, which is good for anti-catabolism and can increase fat burning through thermogenesis. 7-Hydroxy-DHEA is simply a metabolite of 7-Keto-DHEA that is the active form. The two are generally regarded as doing the same things in the body. 7-Keto-DHEA has also shown to promote the immune response when taken orally, giving it many uses for older people looking to keep healthy. Overall, although not a bodybuilding supplement, 7-Keto-DHEA has many benefits, first being increased fat loss and reduced cortisol.

Octopamine - This ingredient has the potential to put on 10-12lbs of lean mass in a 3-4 week period if taken properly. It is not orally bioavailable but sublingually, it should be a very potent muscle producer with some serious mass benefits. Like any other androgen receptor activator, it produces fat loss and weight gain at the same time.

Stacks Cycles and Programs

The different chapters and products have different uses depending on your goals and level of comfort with the ingredients in question. As you move up the stack of ingredients, you are getting progressively more hard core and therefore open to potential side effects. Where Protein and Creatine have little to no issues as far as safety is concerned, we don't recommend that anyone under 18 use anti-estrogens and anyone under 21 use prohormones.

Some good suggestions for the average lifter is to run cycles of these products, adding in some new agents each time to take advantage of the long term genetic changing effects characterized in my book *Change Your Genetics*. By adding in these nutrients and increasing your exposure time, you can rapidly change your basic structure to help your body carry more muscle naturally.

Mixing things like creatine with NO can be accomplished in a variety of products. Then, it is simply a matter of choosing to add in things like pro-hormones and anti-estrogens into the mix. There are many combo products that contain a mix of ingredients detailed in the first few chapters.

A logical progression of utilizing these products would be to follow the natural course laid out in this book, but other variations can be used if one wishes to "jump around" so to speak and get the desired results. Typically, combining the best performers in each category will yield the best results. However, it is possible that a combination of some lesser items will still have good benefits. Some possible combinations of products to help muscle growth and expansion are dependent on many factors, the main one being cash outlay to reach your target goals.

These potential combinations are outlined for your educational purposes only and anything in this book is simply a rough guideline of how to use currently available supplements, it is not an endorsement of any product or combination:

Sample Stack #1:
Natural Stack – Suitable for governed athletes

Protein Supplement
BCAA
Mixed Creatine NO Product
pSARM or Testosterone Building Herbal
GH Releasing Product

Sample Stack #2:
Semi-Natural Stack – Uses your body's own production of testosterone has some ingredients not appropriate for those under 18 or people governed by any athletic body.

Protein Supplement
BCAA
Mixed Creatine / NO Product
Anti-Estrogen

Sample Stack #3:
Prohormone Stack – This is a stack for those over 21 who wish to push their bodies testosterone to levels never before

achieved in sports supplements.
Protein Supplement
BCAA
Mixed / Creatine NO Product
Single Prohormone

Sample Stack #4
Prohormone Super Stack – This stack includes multiple pro-hormones and supporting ingredients and takes hormone production to the highest possible level.

Protein Supplement
BCAA
Mixed Creatine / NO Product
Pro-hormone Stack

Sample Stack #5
Go For Broke Stack – This stack includes all of the above mentioned items and is for people who don't care about cost. The people that use this stack want the best possible results, no matter what the cost and want results that are achievable.

Protein
BCAA
Mixed Creatine / NO Product
Pro-hormone Stack
GH Product At Night
Androgen Receptor Potentiator – Sodium Caprylate
Adaptogen – On training days only or only when fatigued
Stimulant – Pre-workout only

Methyl 1-D

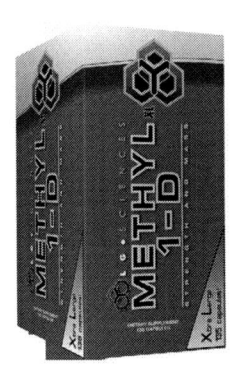

Methyl 1-D contains the only safe and well studied prohormone on the market that is very low on side effects. METHYL 1-D™ is an anabolic animal by itself AND a stack supercharger, too!, which means it can be combined with other prohormones or any sports supplement meant for muscle growth You know that prohormones give you explosive muscle gains and skyrocketing strength that surpass your wildest dreams, which is why Methyl 1-D is the worlds best selling prohormone.

"I'm on my 3rd cycle and I've packed on over 20lbs in total gains! Great product for us hardcore guys"
- Joe T ***results may not be typical*

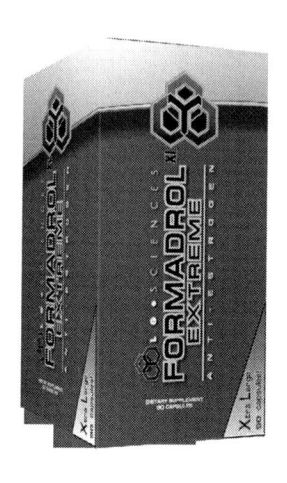

FORMADROL

FORMADROL EXTREME™ ups your Testosterone levels, blocks Estrogen conversion and helps you create your own Testosterone, naturally. ,It's the most powerful Anti-Estrogen, Pro-Testosterone Complex we could find. FORMADROL EXTREME™ combines three ferocious anti-estrogen ingredients absolutely obliterate it while increasing Testosterone at the same time. *"Formadrol made me feel better than any other natural testosterone booster. I actually liked this so much because I leaned out and my sex drive went crazy!" - Adam*

SPEED V2

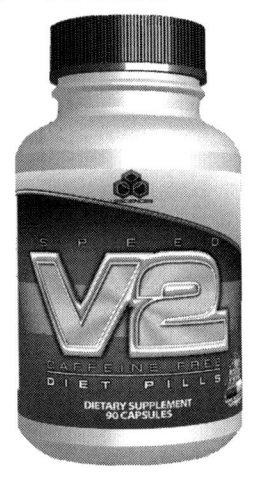

This is the first hardcore diet pill that is 100% caffeine free, but still gives you extra energy and helps reduce appetite better than anything on the market. The key is the synergistic ingredients that ramp up fat burning, reduce appetite and provide complete mental energy.

"I just started taking V2 last week and already I am fitting into my old pants! This product really reduces appetite."

Boris P.

ANADRAULIC STATE

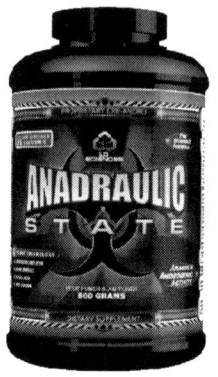

Sometimes a product comes around that takes the supplement world by storm.. Anadraulic State is a preworkout product that combines all the necessary elements to have the perfect workout.

4 NEW TECHNOLOGIES:

S.E.R.M.	AROMATASE INHIBITOR
pSARM	RECEPTOR ENHANCER

IN A BASE OF:

CREATINE	ESSENTIAL AMINO ACIDS
INSULIN MIMETIC	CORTISOL BLOCK

"This stuff is serious. By far the best pre-workout drink I've ever used. Strength, energy, and pumps are out of this world. I am definitely ordering another tub and will run it for 8 weeks. I've told all my gym buddies about this stuff and they are loving it as well. You guys have put together a great product. Thanks again." Matt C.

PERFECT CARB

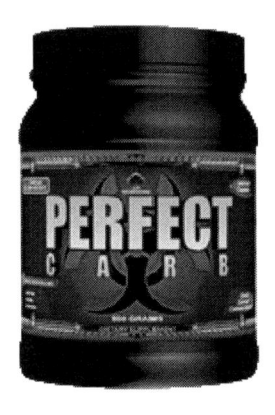

Carbohydrates are important for repair and replenishing muscle glycogen stores. Perfect Carb contains three key nutrients to help boost muscle glycogen stores and increase gastric emptying. Use perfect carb post workout for an instant boost of carbohydrates or add it to your favorite protein drink to make a very effective weight gainer.

BCAA + EAA

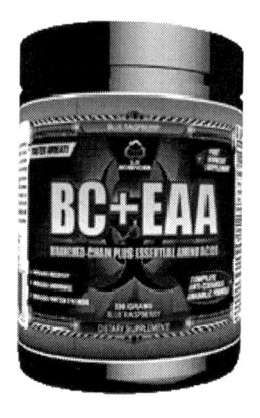

Branched Chain Amino Acids are a staple among bodybuilders for recovery and endurance. High Leucine branched chain amino acids have been shown in scientific literature to increase recovery, induce muscle anabolism and boost nutrient partitioning. We take a very high Leucine, branched chain amino acid mix and then add in hydrolyzed amino acids, which also have been shown in the literature to have a beneficial effect on muscle growth and recovery. This perfect blend tastes great and is best used during workouts or post workout to increase amino acid pools in the bloodstream.

E-911

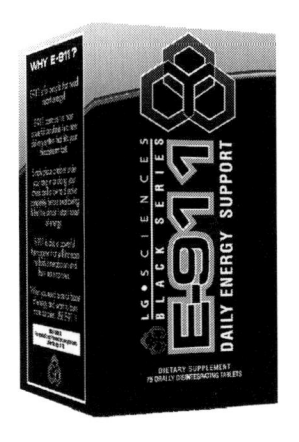

Stimulants are the basis for a good workout. Sadly, it takes a fairly long time for them to enter your blood stream. Luckily with sublingual delivery, it is possible to get immediate impact from this stimulant without the crash associated with swallowed only pill based formulas. E-911 uses three stimulants shown in the literature to boost metabolism and increase thermogenesis, making E-911 an instant hit.